TRENDS AND ADVANCES IN LIVER DISEASES

Liver Regeneration

British Library Cataloguing in Publication Data
A catalogue record for this book is available from the British Library.

ISBN 086196-347-4

Éditions John Libbey Eurotext
6, rue Blanche, 92120 Montrouge, France.
Tél. : (1) 47.35.85.52 – Fax : (1) 46.57.10.09

John Libbey and Company Ltd
13, Smith Yard, Summerley Street, London SW18 4HR, England
Tél. : (81) 947.27.77

John Libbey CIC
Via L. Spallanzani, 11
00161, Rome, Italy
Tél. : (06) 862.289

© 1992, Paris

Il est interdit de reproduire intégralement ou partiellement le présent ouvrage – loi du 11 mars 1957 – sans autorisation de l'éditeur ou du Centre Français du Copyright, 6 *bis* rue Gabriel Laumain, 75010 Paris, France.

TRENDS AND ADVANCES IN LIVER DISEASES

Liver Regeneration

Proceedings of the International Congress
held in Gouvieux-Chantilly (France)
February, 7-8, 1992

Editors

D. Bernuau
G. Feldmann

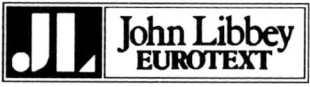

TRENDS AND ADVANCES IN LIVER DISEASES
The first volume of this series was published in September 1991
Immunological, metabolic and infectious aspects of liver transplantation
D.A. Vuitton, C. Balabaud, D. Houssin, D. Dhumeaux
1991, paperback, 120 pages, 165 F.

This book has been published
with the cooperation of Roche Laboratories.

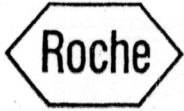

Contents

List of contributors VII
Foreword IX

Liver regeneration : models and mechanisms. *N. Fausto (Providence, USA)* 1

Morphological estimation of liver cell regeneration. *G. Feldmann (Paris, France)* 7

Liver stem cells : myth or reality ? *J.Y. Scoazec (Paris, France)* 17

Role of sinusoidal cells in liver regeneration. *P. Bioulac-Sage, L. Dubuisson, B. Le Bail, P. Bernard, J. Carles, P. Lefebvre, C. Balabaud (Bordeaux, France)* 29

Ito cell proliferation *in vivo* and *in vitro*. *J. Rosenbaum, F. Charlotte (Créteil, France)* 39

Cyclin A and liver cell proliferation. *F. Zindy, J. Wang, E. Lamas, X. Chenivesse, B. Henglein, C. Bréchot (Paris, France)* 49

Cell cycle progression of adult rat hepatocytes *in vitro*. *P. Loyer, D. Glaise, L. Meijer, C. Guguen-Guillouzo (Rennes, France)* 61

Oncogenes and liver regeneration. *J. Sobczak (Paris, France)* 71

Regulation of liver growth by transforming growth factor alpha. *N. Fausto (Providence, USA)* 77

Hepatocyte growth factor (HGF). *G.K. Michalopoulos, R. Zarnegar, R. Appasamy (Pittsburgh, USA)* 85

Insulin-like growth factor II (IGF-II) in human primary liver cancer : a progression factor and/or a marker of liver cell differentiation. *C. Bréchot, F. Zindy, E. Cariani, E. Lamas, C. Lasserre (Paris, France)* 103

Contents

Alpha-fetoprotein and hepatocyte proliferation.
D. Bernuau, I. Tournier, J.Y. Scoazec, G. Feldmann (Paris, France) 117

The role of growth limiting mechanisms in the regulation of liver mass and liver regeneration. *C. Nadal (Orsay, France)* 123

Proliferative responsiveness of human hepatocytes in culture : evidence for the transitory expression of hepatotrophic factor(s) in the serum of patients with fulminant hepatitis or after partial hepatectomy.
P. Blanc, H. Etienne, M. Daujat, I. Fabre, J. Domergue, C. Astre, B. Saint Aubert, H. Michel, P. Maurel (Montpellier, France) 129

Liver regeneration : the surgeon's point of view.
Y. Panis, J. Belghiti (Clichy, France) 139

Fulminant and subfulminant hepatitis : liver regeneration and prognosis.
J. Bernuau (Clichy, France) 147

Author Index 159

Key word Index 161

List of contributors

Bernuau D. *et al.*, Laboratoire de Biologie Cellulaire, INSERM U.327, Faculté de Médecine Xavier Bichat, 16 rue Henri Huchard, 75018 Paris, France.

Bernuau J., Service d'Hépatologie, Hôpital Beaujon, 100 Boulevard du Général Leclerc, 92210 Clichy, France.

Bioulac-Sage P. *et al.*, Laboratoire des Interactions Cellulaires, Université Bordeaux II, 146 rue Léo-Saignat, 33076 Bordeaux Cedex, France.

Blanc P. *et al.*, INSERM U.128, CNRS, Route de Mende, BP 5051, 34033 Montpellier Cedex, France.

Bréchot C. *et al.*, INSERM U.75, Faculté de Médecine Necker, 156 rue de Vaugirard, 75730 Paris Cedex 15, France.

Fausto N., Department of Pathology and Laboratory Medicine, Division of Biology and Medicine, Box G, Providence RI 02912, USA.

Feldmann G., Laboratoire de Biologie Cellulaire, INSERM U.327, Faculté de Médecine Xavier Bichat, 16 rue Henri Huchard, 75018 Paris, France.

Loyer P. *et al.*, INSERM U.49, Hôpital de Pontchaillou, Rue Henri le Guilloux, 35033 Rennes Cedex, France.

Michalopoulos G.K. *et al.*, Department of Pathology, University of Pittsburgh, School of Medicine, 718 Scaife Hall, Pittsburgh PA 15261, USA.

Nadal C., URA 1343 du CNRS, Institut Curie, Section de Biologie, Centre Universitaire, 91405 Orsay Cedex, France.

Panis Y. and Belghiti J., Service de Chirurgie Digestive, Hôpital Beaujon, 100 boulevard du Général Leclerc, 92110 Clichy, France.

Rosenbaum J. and Charlotte F., INSERM U.99, Hôpital Henri Mondor, 51 Avenue du Maréchal de Lattre de Tassigny, 94010 Créteil, France.

Scoazec J.Y., Laboratoire de Biologie Cellulaire, INSERM U.327, Faculté de Médecine Xavier Bichat, 16 rue Henri Huchard, 75018 Paris, France.

Sobczak J., Faculté de Médecine Necker, INSERM U.75, Service de Biochimie, 156 rue de Vaugirard, 75472 Paris Cedex 15, France.

Zindy F. *et al.*, INSERM U.75, Faculté de Médecine Necker, 156 rue de Vaugirard, 75730 Paris Cedex 15, France.

Foreword

In the series of seminars organized by the French Association for the Study of the Liver, a meeting on "Liver Regeneration" has been held in Gouvieux-Chantilly (France), on February 7th and 8th 1992. The success of such seminars, whose aim is to bring together in an informal manner basic liver cell biologists and hepatologists, is now well confirmed, and has been particularly obvious at Gouvieux-Chantilly.
Liver regeneration is a fascinating aspect of liver physiology, involving numerous developing fields of modern cell biology, such as regulation of the cell cycle, growth factors and oncogenes. The seminar at Chantilly has provided a comprehensive view of these various factors, and the possible implications in the pathogenesis of hepatocarcinoma have been approached.
We thank all the lecturers for their active contribution which has made possible the realisation of this book, Mrs Bedin and Centonze for the material organization of the meeting, and John Libbey Eurotext for accepting to publish for the second time a book on the seminar in the series of "Trends and Advances in Liver Diseases".

D. Bernuau
G. Feldmann

Liver regeneration : models and mechanisms

Nelson Fausto

Department of Pathology and Laboratory Medicine, Brown University, Providence, Rhode Island 02912, USA

The liver has a remarkable capacity to regulate its growth and size as demonstrated by the restoration of liver mass that occurs after partial hepatectomy in humans and animals. Liver regeneration is a strictly regulated, non-autonomous process controlled by positive and negative factors which ultimately act to reestablish the appropriate ratio between liver mass and body size (Fausto, 1990). Growth ends when the original liver mass is regained through hyperplasia of the cells in the lobes of the liver remnant (compensatory growth).

The knowledge acquired from work on liver regeneration in animals has proven to be directly applicable to studies involving transplanted human livers and partially hepatectomized patients (Nagasue et al., 1987). One of the most striking demonstrations of hepatic growth regulation in humans is the observation that transplanted livers which are small for a host will grow until the organ reaches the optimal mass required for this person (VanThiel et al., 1987). This finding has led to the use of split transplants and the increased utilization of living donor transplantation (Strong et al., 1990; Broelsch et al., 1990). In this latter situation, the liver remnant in the partially hepatectomized donor, as well as the liver transplanted into the new host, grow until they reach the hepatic mass which is appropriate for each of these individuals.

In humans and animals, excess hepatic functional capacity, if established, does not persist and is quickly corrected by tissue atrophy or cell loss. Examples of this type of adaptation are the lack of growth and decrease in size of a transplant that is large for the new host (Kam et al., 1987) and the rapid loss of cells (presumably by apoptosis) that occurs in hypertrophic normal livers when the source of the growth stimulus is removed (Mead et al., 1990). An interesting situation is encountered in human heterotopic liver transplantation. In these cases, loss of function and atrophy of the natural liver quickly accelerates after transplantation (Willemse et al., 1992). In the few described cases in which the natural liver regains its function (sometimes 1-2 years after the transplant operation) it is the heterotopically transplanted liver which undergoes atrophy (Metselaar et al., 1990). Thus, a process of apparent "functional competition" between natural and transplanted liver takes place and leads to the survival of either one but not of both livers.

The central problem that emerges from these general considerations on liver growth regulation is to know how the optimal functional mass of the liver is established and maintained. It is apparent that optimal mass is maintained by a dynamic equilibrium between body demands and liver function. Although the adult liver is a non-proliferative organ, a disruption of the equilibrium leads to the initiation of a compensatory growth response which lasts until the original liver mass is restored. The signals for the initiation and termination of the process are likely to be related to hepatic function rather than anatomical form because growth of the liver remnant occurs without regeneration of the lobes removed at the operation (Fausto and Mead, 1989).

Models of liver regeneration

A number of models can be proposed to explain how optimal hepatic functional mass is reestablished after partial hepatectomy. These models are based on 3 general assumptions: a) that liver growth is related to liver function; b) that hepatic growth regulation depends on interactions between circulating (endocrine) factors and those produced in liver tissue (autocrine and paracrine factors); c) that liver growth regulation relies on positive and negative signals that trigger, modulate and stop the process. The 3 models that I will propose differ mostly in assigning an active or a passive (target) role for the liver in the regenerative response (Fig 1). Model 1 is based on the notion that there is a linkage between functional demands on the liver and the initiation of the events that lead to hepatocyte DNA replication. The exact nature of the link is not clear but a series of reasonable hypotheses can be made. It is conceivable that hepatocyte entry into the cell cycle (Go/G1 transition) may be mediated by the increased load imposed on the liver remnant to maintain normal metabolic functions. Many rapid metabolic adaptations occur in the first 2 hours after partial hepatectomy, as indicated by changes in liver electrolyte concentrations and the accumulation of amino acids which are components of the urea cycle (Bucher and Malt, 1971; Short et al., 1973)). Other experiments show that nutritional changes (amino acid overload preceded by a short period of protein deprivation) in intact non-hepatectomized rats can trigger the activation of immediate early genes in a pattern that may mimic the sequence of events that take place during the first few hours after partial hepatectomy (Bucher et al., 1978; Horikawa et al., 1986; Mead et al., 1990). The increase in steady-state levels of mRNA from these genes (and presumably the elevation of their protein products) is associated with the entry of hepatocytes into the cell cycle ("priming"). However, "primed" hepatocytes do not by themselves progress through the cell cycle (G1 to S) but instead require stimulation by growth factors such as TGFα. One possibility is that the quiescent hepatocyte in Go does not respond to this factor but cells in early G1 acquire the capacity to respond. This two stage model of hepatocyte replication (requiring priming followed by progression) places equal emphasis on triggering of the Go/G1 transition and in the steps that make the primed hepatocytes progress from G1 to S. Both of these events may be key regulatory points in controlling hepatocyte replication after partial hepatectomy (Fausto and Mead, 1989).

Model number 2 assumes that liver growth is regulated by the level of a serum factor which is a hepatic mitogen (Fig 1).. Under normal conditions, the concentration of the circulating factor would be too low to cause hepatocyte replication. However, when the levels of the factor rise above a certain threshold, a proliferative response that leads to DNA replication is initiated. The conditions that may cause the blood concentration of the factor to increase above the mitogenic threshold depend on the nature and site of production of the factor. Thus, if under normal conditions there is active hepatic uptake of a factor produced in other tissues, blood concentrations of the substance might increase as a consequence of liver injury or decreased cell mass. Conceivably, blood accumulation of the factor could also occur even when the liver is intact, as long as the production of the factor in extrahepatic sites exceeds liver uptake. On the other hand, if the blood mitogen is mostly synthesized in the liver and from there released into the circulation, cell injury and death of hepatic cells could cause an eleva-

Models of Liver Regeneration

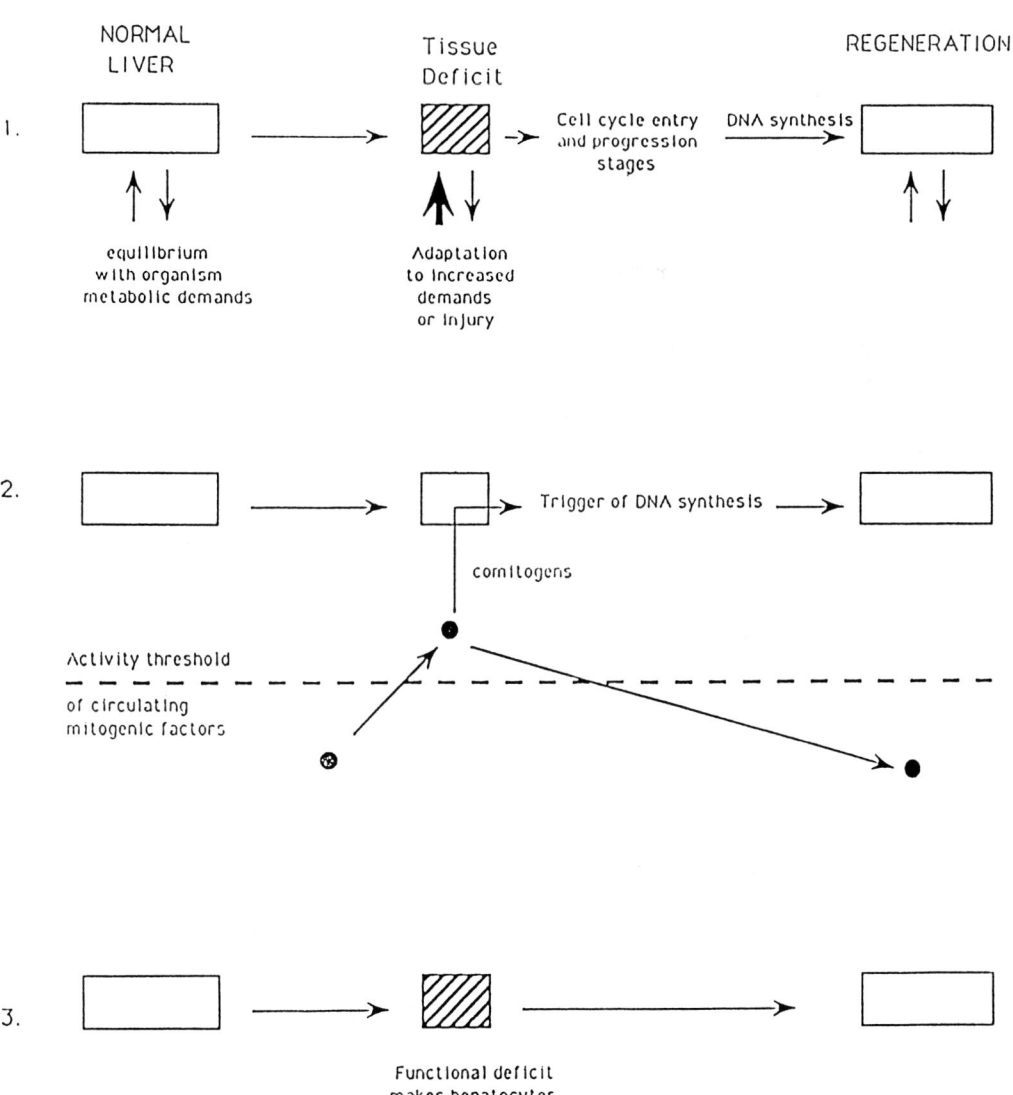

Figure 1

tion in blood levels. The mechanism for this type of increase might be similar to the release of transaminases into the serum after hepatocyte injury or could involve modulations of gene expression similar to those observed during the acute phase response. In this model, the liver serves as a target for a circulating mitogen and has essentially a passive role in the growth process. The model implies (although this is not an obligatory requirement) that the key control for the growth response lies in the initiating stage. Further, the model predicts that a significant level of hepatocyte replication in the normal liver can be achieved by injection or infusion of the factor. The only known factor that can fulfill the role of the circulating hepatic mitogen required by this model is HGF (Michalopoulos, 1990; 1992). Future work should show whether HGF is released from hepatic tissue in liver injury, if its uptake is decreased after partial hepatectomy or toxic injury and whether its production is modulated in other tissues in connection with alterations of the functional mass of the liver (Kinoshita, 1991).

Model 3 combines the main features of the two previous models (Fig 1). It assumes that after partial hepatectomy there are changes in hepatocytes (perhaps induced by functional demands) which make them capable of responding to mitogenic factors, either circulating or produced in liver tissue.

Negative controls

All of the models discussed so far rely exclusively on the action of positive stimuli, that is, growth factors which are complete mitogens for hepatocytes in primary culture. However, it is most likely that negative regulators may be of equal importance as the positive stimulators. The negative regulators are inhibitors of hepatocyte replication *in vitro* (and most likely *in vivo*) and their absolute concentrations (or the ratio between positive/negative effectors) may need to increase to permit hepatocyte proliferation and to decrease to terminate growth. The whole issue may be approached from a more general perspective by asking whether hepatocyte replication in the normal liver is held in check by the presence of mitotic inhibitors. A strong argument in favor of the existence of inhibitors is the difficulty of inducing hepatocyte proliferation in normal intact livers. Furthermore, although hepatocytes isolated from fetal livers or newborn rats can replicate to some extent in culture in absence of serum or growth factors, adult hepatocytes display minimal replicative capacity in culture, even in rich medium, as long as a growth factors (EGF/TGFα, HGF etc.) or serum are not added (McGowan, 1986). This suggests that if inhibitors of hepatocyte proliferation play a physiological role in maintaining the low proliferative state of normal adult hepatocytes, these factors might be produced by hepatocytes themselves.

TGFβ1 is the best characterized inhibitor of hepatocyte DNA synthesis although various laboratories are actively involved in the purification of other inhibitory substances (see Nadal, this volume). The major puzzles regarding the anti-mitogenic effects of TGFβ in the liver have not been solved and may be summarized as follows: a) the liver contains TGFβ1,2, and 3, all of which inhibit hepatocyte DNA replication and are produced by non-parenchymal cells; b) levels of TGFβ mRNAs increase after partial hepatectomy; c) the kinetics of the increase differs among members of the family and mRNA elevation occurs quite early and transiently (4-8 h after partial hepatectomy followed by a decrease) for TGFβ2 and β3 mRNAs; d) although maximal increases in TGFβ1 mRNA occur after the major wave of DNA replication, mRNA levels are higher than normal throughout the prereplicative stage that precedes DNA synthesis; e) the ratios between active TGFβ and the latent complex in hepatic tissue during liver regeneration are not known (Braun *et al.*, 1988; Jakowlew *et al.*, 1991; Nakatsukasa *et al.*, 1990). Thus, rather than decreasing during the growth process as would be expected of an inhibitor of hepatocyte DNA synthesis, TGFβ1 increases in the regenerating liver and we do not know why 3 TGFβ forms with the same apparent effects and the same cellular distribution are needed. A major problem in dealing with this issue is the lack of data on the amounts of active TGFβ peptides found in resting and growing hepatic tissue. Until answers to these questions are obtained, it is difficult to assess the physiological role of TGFβ1 in preventing or terminating hepatocyte replication.

Although we generally think of inhibitory signals as being provided by growth factors (through a paracrine effect in the case of TGFβs and hepatocytes) the same type of inhibition may be accomplished by the expression in hepatocytes of suppressor genes which inhibit one or more stages of the cell cycle. One of the best candidates for this role is the retinoblastoma gene (Rb) which undergoes changes in phosphorylation levels as cells progress in the cell cycle (DeCaprio et al., 1992).

Strategies for the study of liver regeneration

The main focus of studies of mechanisms of liver regeneration has gone through phases that emphasized in succession, morphology, physiology and biochemistry. At the present time heavy reliance has been placed on molecular biology. From this perspective, fruitful areas of research include among others, work on protooncogenes and suppressor genes, transcriptional factors, growth factors and receptors, cell cycle components and cell and matrix interactions. As exciting as these topics are, it is evident that the detailed analysis of each of them in isolation, although essential, will not be sufficient to provide a clear understanding of liver regeneration. Liver growth responses involve the whole organ and the totality of its cellular, matrix and vascular components. The real understanding of hepatic growth regulation requires the analysis of how these various compartments interact and how each cell type produces factors and reacts to stimuli generated by other hepatic cells or in extrahepatic sites. It is however a very hopeful trend, that in conjunction with molecular biology approaches, studies of liver growth in clinical settings involving transplantation, partial hepatectomy or recovery after injury are receiving increased attention. The clinical work has benefited from the knowledge acquired with experimental systems and at the same time has provided new insights and hypotheses that can be tested in animal experiments. These combined approaches hold great promise for the future.

REFERENCES

Bucher, N.L.R. and Malt, R.A. (1971): Regeneration of the liver and kidney. Boston: Little Brown.
Bucher, N.L.R., McGowan, J.A. and Patel, U. (1978): Hormonal regulation of liver growth. ICN/UCLA Symposium on Molecular and Cell Biology 12, 661-670.
Braun, L., Mead, J.E., Panzica, M., Mikumo, R., Bell, G.I. and Fausto, N. (1988): Elevation of transforming growth factor-beta mRNA during liver regeneration: A possible paracrine mechanism of growth regulation. Proc. Natl. Acad. Sci. U.S.A. 85, 1534-1538.
Broelsch, C.E., Emond, J.C., Whitington, P.F., Thistlethwaite, J.R., Baker, A.L. and Lichtor, J.L. (1990): Application of reduced-size liver transplants as split grafts, auxiliary orthotopic grafts, and living related segmental transplants. Ann. Surg. 212, 368-375.
DeCaprio, J.A., Furukawa, Y., Ajchenbaum, F., Griffin, J.D. and Livingston, D.M. (1992): The retinoblastoma-susceptibility gene product becomes phosphorylated in multiple stages during cell cycle entry and progression. Proc. Natl. Acad. Sci. U.S.A. 89, 1795-1798.
Fausto, N. (1990): Hepatic regeneration. In Hepatology: A textbook of liver disease, ed. D. Zakim and T.D. Boyer, pp 49-62. Philadelphia: W.B. Saunders.

Fausto, N. and Mead, J.E. (1989). Regulation of liver growth: protooncogenes and transforming growth factors. *Lab. Invest.* 60, 4-13.

Horikawa, S., Sakata, K., Hatanaka, M. and Tsukada, K. (1986): Expression of c-myc oncogene in rat liver by a dietary manipulation. *Biochem. Biophys. Res. Commun.* 140, 574-580.

Jakowlew, S.B., Mead, J.E., Danielpour, D., Wu, J., Roberts, A.B. and Fausto, N. (1991): Transforming growth factor-β (TGF-β) isoforms in rat liver regeneration: messenger RNA expression and activation of latent TGFβ. *Cell Regulation* 2, 535-548.

Kam, I., Lynch, S., Svanas, G., Todo, S., Polimeno, L., Francavilla, A., Penkrot, R.J., Takaya, S., Ericzon, B.G., Starzl, T.E. and Van Thiel, D.H. (1987): Evidence that host size determines liver size: studies in dogs receiving orthotopic liver transplants. *Hepatology* 7, 362-366.

Kinoshita, T., Hirao, S., Matsumoto, K. and Nakamura, T. (1991): Possible endocrine control by hepatocyte growth factor of liver regeneration after partial hepatectomy. *Biochem. Biophys. Res. Commun.* 177, 330-335.

McGowan, J.A. (1986): Hepatocyte proliferation in culture. In *Research in isolated and cultured hepatocytes*, ed. A. Guillouzo and C. Guguen-Guillouzo, pp 259-283. London: John Libbey Co.

Mead, J.E., Braun, L., Martin, D.A. and Fausto, N. (1990): Induction of replicative competence ("priming") in normal liver. *Cancer Res.* 50, 7023-7030.

Metselaar, H.J., Hesselink, E.J., deRave, S., ten Kate, F.J.W., Lameris, J.S., Groenland, T.H.N., Revvers, C.B., Weimar, W., Terpstra, O.T. and Schalm, S.W. (1990): Recovery of failing liver after auxiliary heterotopic transplantation. *The Lancet* 335, 1156-1157.

Michalopoulos, G.K. (1990): Liver regeneration: molecular mechanisms of growth control. *FASEB J.* 4, 176-187.

Michalopoulos, G.K. (1992): Hepatocyte growth factor. *Hepatology* 15, 149-155.

Nagasue, N., Yukaya, H., Ogawa, Y., Kohno, H. and Nakamura, T. (1987): Human liver regeneration after major hepatic resection. A study of normal liver and liver with chronic hepatitis and cirrhosis. *Ann. Surg.* 206, 30-39.

Nakatsukasa, H., Evarts, R.P., Hsia, C-C. and Thorgeirsson, S.S. (1990): Transforming growth factor β1 and Type I procollagen transcripts during regeneration and early fibrosis of rat liver. *Lab. Invest.* 63, 171-180.

Short, J., Armstrong, N.B., Zemel, R. and Lieberman, I. (1973): A role for amino acids in the induction of deoxyribonucleic acid synthesis in liver. *Biochem. Biophys. Res. commun.* 50, 430-437.

Strong, R.W., Lynch, S.V., Ong, T.H., Matsunami, H., Koido, Y. and Balderson, G.A. (1990): Successful liver transplantation from a living donor to her son. *New England J. Med.* 322: 1505-1507.

Van Thiel, D.H., Gavaler, J.S., Kam, I., Francavilla, A., Polimeno, L., Schade, R.R., Smith, J., Diven, W., Penkrot, R.J. and Starzl, T.E. (1987): Rapid growth of an intact human liver transplanted into recipient larger than the donor. *Gastroenterology* 93: 1414-1419.

Willemse, P.J.A., Ausema, L., Terpstra, O.T., Krenning, E.P., ten Kate, F.W.J. and Schalam, S. (1992): Graft regeneration and host liver atrophy after auxiliary heterotopic liver transplantation for chronic liver failure. *Hepatology* 15, 54-57.

Liver Regeneration. Eds D. Bernuau, G. Feldmann. John Libbey Eurotext, Paris © 1992, pp. 7-16.

Morphological estimation of liver cell regeneration

Gérard Feldmann

INSERM U.327, Laboratoire de Biologie Cellulaire, Faculté de Médecine Xavier Bichat, 16 rue Henri Huchard, 75018 Paris, France

INTRODUCTION

Like for other cells, liver cell regeneration is accompanied by morphological changes in the cytoplasm and nucleus of hepatic cells (Martin et Feldmann, 1983). Cytoplasmic changes take the appearance of subttle modifications of some organelles such as the ribosomes, the glycogen particles or the plasma membrane. For instance, regeneration of hepatocytes is given to be characterized by an increase in the number of bound ribosomes, the clustering of glycogen particles leading to formation of glycogenic bodies or the appearance of microvilli all along the plasma membrane (Phillips et al, 1987). None of these alterations is specific and their link to the regenerative process of hepatocytes remains to be demonstrated. Such situation exists also for the other hepatic cells, the sinusoidal and biliary cells, where cytoplasmic changes indicating a possible regeneration are uneasy to recognize.

In fact the best way to appreciate liver cell regeneration is to look at mitoses in the liver. However, search for mitoses is time-consuming, particularly because in the normal liver the percentage of dividing liver cells is very low (Fabrikant, 1968) and also because the recognition of mitoses is not so easy in pathological processes where liver architecture is deeply disturbed. In addition, mitosis represents only a small part of the cell cycle. For instance in the rat liver, the mitotic phase is estimated to be of about 1 hour (Edwards and Koch, 1964 ; Barbason and Van Cantfort, 1976), a normal hepatocyte cycle being of 24 hours (Fabrikant, 1968) with approximately 8 hours for the S phase (Edwards and Koch, 1964). If we add that the mean life-span of hepatocytes is given to be around 300 days in the adult rat (MacDonald, 1961), chances to observe a dividing cell in the normal liver are very rare. Consequently investigation of the other parts of the cell cycle which are longer that the M phase, is very interesting since it can complete our information on liver cell regeneration. At the present time, many markers are available to analyse the different phases of the cell cycle. Some of them are commonly used or begin to be used in liver cell regeneration. Others are also possible to study the cell cycle but are not employed at the present time in liver cell regeneration.
The aim of this review is to discuss the advantages and inconvenients of the markers commonly employed to investigate liver cell regeneration.

MARKERS COMMONLY USED IN LIVER CELL REGENERATION

A) Tritiated thymidine

[3H] thymidine, a marker of the S phase, the DNA-synthetizing phase or replicative phase, is the oldest morphological marker used in liver cell regeneration. It has been proposed at least 30 years ago to measure the cell cycle of hepatocytes in normal rat liver and in regenerating rat liver after partial hepatectomy (MacDonald, 1961 ; Grisham, 1962; Fabrikant, 1968). [3H] thymidine can be used either *in vivo* or *in vitro* . *In vivo*, preparation of animals, most often the rats, is the following : a single dose with variable amounts of [3H] thymidine, between 0.2 mCi (Grisham, 1962) to 1 mCi (Geerts et al, 1991) per kg/body weight, is administered intraperitoneally or sometimes intraveinously to the animal, 1 or 2h before the sacrifice of the animal. Repeated or continuous administration and in the last case with the use of a subcutaneous pump (Eldridge et al, 1990), are also possible . After the sacrifice, liver fragments are processed according to routine histological techniques. Briefly they are fixed in 10 % neutral formalin or in a mixture of alcohol, formalin, acetic acid, dehydrated and embedded in paraffin. Autohistoradiography is made on liver sections. An exposure time of 2 to 3 weeks is in general sufficient but depends on the dose and specific activity of the isotope. After autohistoradiography sections can be stained with hematoxylin and eosin. Labelling index (number of positive nuclei per 1000 cells) is counted on light microscopy. Control reactions are made with rats not receiving [3H] thymidine and liver sections prepared according to the same procedure.

Using this technique, several authors have established some data which are now well accepted. In the rat, the labelling index of regenerating hepatocytes is at it maximum 24 hours after partial hepatectomy, i.e. about 40 % (Grisham, 1962 ; Fabrikant, 1968 ; Rabes, 1976). The maximum for sinusoidal cells is observed between 42 to 50 hours (Grisham, 1962 ; Fabrikant, 1968) and is of 30 %. In contrast in the normal rat liver the percentage of [3H] thymidine positive-cells is of 0.3 % for the hepatocytes and 0.9 % for sinusoidal cells. It has been also established by the same authors that after hepatectomy, hepatocyte regeneration begins in the periportal zone of the hepatic lobule, then progressively extends to the medio and centrolobular zones to be roughly equal in the 3 zones at the begining of the third day after hepatectomy.

In vitro, [3H] thymidine is also very often used to appreciate the role of factors acting on the hepatic cell cycle and the effects of the numerous drugs which are metabolized by the hepatic cells. The technique is similar to that used *in vivo*. After plating, primary cultures of rat hepatocytes are incubated for 60 min with [3H] thymidine at 37° C under an atmosphere of 95% air, 5 % CO_2. We used in our laboratory a concentration of 2.5 mCi per ml/l but lower concentrations are possible (Sand et al, 1989. Tomomura et al, 1987 ; Martin et al, 1991). Longer incubations (24 hours) are also proposed. After incubation, hepatic cells are fixed in buffered formalin, or in a mixture of alcohol and acetic acid. Autohistoradiography is performed on the plates themselves and the labelling index is counted, generally after an exposure time of 2 weeks but, like *in vivo* this time depends on the dose and activity of the isotope. Results are given in Fig. 1.

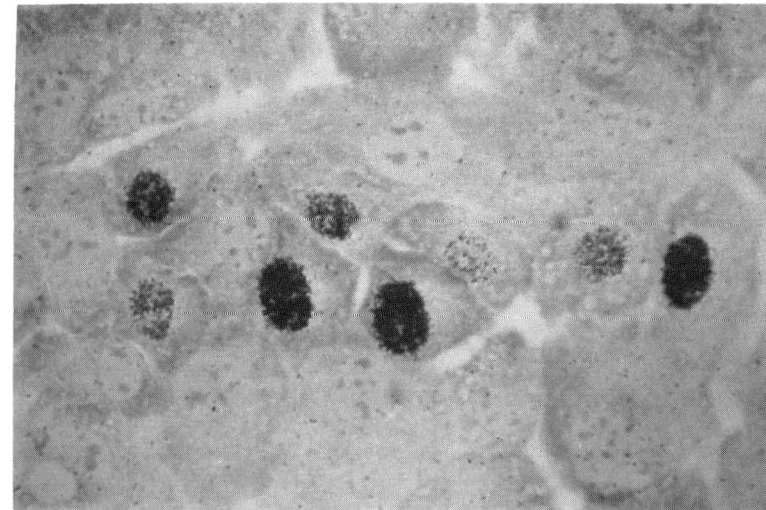

Fig. 1 : Primary cultures of rat hepatocytes. [3H] thymidine is visible in the nuclei of some hepatocytes

[^{3}H] thymidine is very rarely used to investigate liver cell regeneration in human liver. However one example is provided by Leevy (1963) who proposed to incubate human liver fragments immediately after their obtention by needle biopsy, in a Ringer solution containing [^{3}H] thymidine (0.15 mCi/ml) for 90 min at 37°C in a water-bath shaker under a controled O^2 (95%), CO^2 (5%) atmosphere. Autohistoradiography was performed on liver sections after fixation and embedding of liver fragments according to routine histological techniques. Results obtained by this author are difficult to interpret : in general a very low percentage of [^{3}H] thymidine-positive hepatic cells was observed, whatever was the pathological situation investigated (viral hepatitis, fatty liver, alcoholic cirrhosis), this percentage being between 0.02 % and 0.12 % of all the hepatic cells. Moreover, no significant difference was recorded in the different clinical forms of hepatitis (acute *versus* chronic hepatitis) or in alcoholic *versus* non alcoholic cirrhosis. It is probably these disappointing results which discouraged the others researchers to use [^{3}H] thymidine to investigate regeneration in human liver fragments.

To conclude with [^{3}H] thymidine it must be stressed that the technique presents some obvious advantages : it is well standardized, well reproductible and easy to perform. We can add that the nuclear labelling is easy to recognize and that the development of automatic image analysers can greatly facilitate the measure of the labeling index. In contrast [^{3}H] thymidine presents two inconvenients : use of radioactive isotopes and a long exposure time.

B) Bromodeoxyuridine

The 5'-bromo-2'-deoxyuridine (BrdU) is a thymidine analogue which incorporates in DNA-synthetizing cells during the S phase of the cell cycle. Its use in the investigation of replicating cells became possible when monoclonal antibodies against BrdU were available (Gratzner, 1982). A symposium summarizing the conditions of using monoclonal antibodies against BrdU was published in 1985 (Gray and Mayall, 1985). Like [^{3}H] thymidine, BrdU can be used *in vivo* or *in vitro*.

In vivo, preparation of the animals is simple : a single dose of BrdU, between 50 to 200 mg/kg/body weight (Eldridge et al, 1990 ; deFazio et al, 1987 ; Frederiks et al, 1990 ; Tanaka et al, 1990 ; Paolucci et al, 1990), is injected intraperitoneally or sometimes intravenously to the animals which are sacrificed 1 or 2 hours after the injection. Continuous administration of BrdU with a subcutaneous pump is also proposed (Eldridge et al, 1990). The preparation of tissue fragments has been studied extensively (Schutte et al, 1987). Liver fragments can be either fixed in various fixatives or immediately frozen in liquid nitrogen and stored at -80°C. The choice of the fixative is important. For instance, Schutte et al (1987), have observed that the immunoreactivity of BrdU in the mouse small intestine varied according to the fixative. Immunoreactivity was better when the tissue was fixed in formalin or Carnoy's fluid than in Bouin's fluid or in a mixture of paraformaldehyde and lysine. No reactivity was observed when the intestine was fixed in glutaraldehyde or in the lysine-periodate-paraformaldehyde fixative. Finally, the reactivity was good when the tissue was frozen only. After fixation, cryostat or paraffin sections are made according to the initial choice.

Before incubation of the sections with monoclonal anti-BrdU antibodies, denaturation of the double-stranded DNA is absolutely necessary. Most often, this denaturation is obtained by incubating sections with HCl. Slight variations regarding the acid concentration, temperature and incubation time are described (Eldridge et al 1990 ; deFazio et al, 1987 ; Frederiks et al, 1990 ; Schutte et al 1987 ; Shimizu et al, 1988 ; Tanaka et al, 1990) ; generally HCl is used at a concentration varying from 1 N to 4 N, at a temperature of 37°C or 40°C with an incubation time between 20 to 60 min. Formamide can sometimes replace HCl (Paolucci et al, 1990). A proteolytic digestion with pepsine or pronase can be added to the denaturation step. For instance, Schutte et al (1987) have observed that tissue digestion with pepsin, before acid denaturation, increased remarkably the immunoreactivity of BrdU when the tissue was fixed with glutaraldehyde. Monoclonal antibodies against BrdU are commercially available. An indirect immunohistochemical method is used, the second antibody being labelled with peroxidase or alkaline phosphatase. Biotinylated mouse immunoglobulins and avidin-biotin-peroxidase complex can also be used. After histochemical demonstration of peroxidase or alkaline phosphatase, liver sections are examined on light microscopy. Most often the intensity of the reaction is sufficient and no other staining is necessary. A labelling index per 1000 hepatocytes or sinusoidal cells is measured. Automatic image analyser can be employed since the product of the histochemical reaction, brown for peroxidase or red for alkaline phosphatase is easily recognized by the analyser. Control reactions can be made by preparing control rats not receiving BrdU or by incubating the liver sections with the second antibody only.

Using BrdU incorporation, results obtained in the rat with [^{3}H] thymidine in liver cell regeneration after partial hepatectomy have been confirmed. Twenty-four hours after the operation, the percentage of BrdU positive-hepatocytes was of 36 % (Frederiks et al, 1990) while the maximum observed for Ito cells, one of the sinusoidal cell, was of 25 % (Tanaka et al, 1990) 48 h after hepatectomy. These two values are roughly similar to that obtained by Grisham (1962) , Fabrikant (1968) and Rabes (1976) with [^{3}H] thymidine. Values obtained in incorporating BrdU in normal rat liver are also very low.

BrdU incorporation is also used to appreciate liver cell regeneration *in vitro*. Several protocols are used. For instance, we use the following in our laboratory : after plating, primary cultures of rat hepatocytes are incubated for 1 or 2 hr at 37°C with a solution of BrdU (10 mg/ml) under a 95 % air, 5% CO_2 atmosphere. After washing, cultures are fixed in a mixture of alcohol and acetic acid. Denaturation of double -stranded DNA can be made with formamide or HCl. Cells are permeabilized with a solution of 0.1% Triton X100 and incubated with monoclonal anti-BrdU antibodies. The following steps are similar to those used for *in vivo* BrdU incorporation. Results are given in Fig.2.

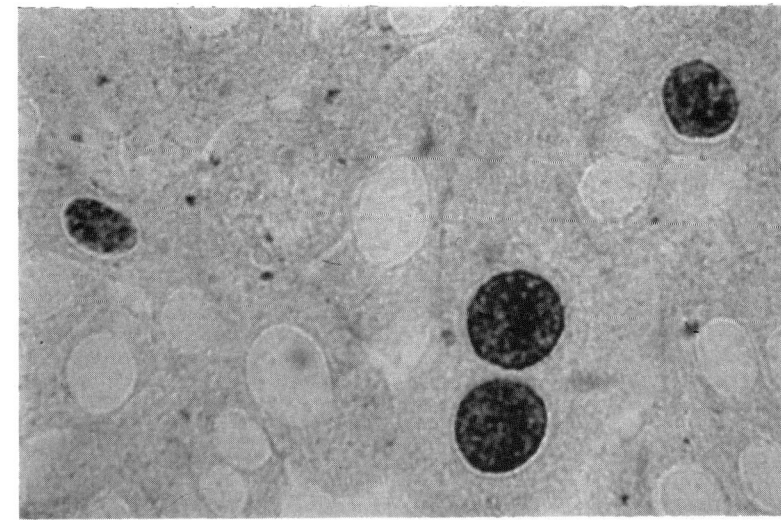

Fig. 2 : Primary cultures of rat hepatocytes. Bromodeoxyuridine is visible in the nuclei of some hepatocytes

Recently, a technique has been proposed to measure liver cell regeneration by incorporating BrdU in human liver fragments obtained by needle biopsy (Shimizu et al, 1988 ; Tarao et al, 1991). Liver specimens are incubated for 45 min in a solution of 0.1% BrdU in RPMI 1640 at 37°C in a water-bath shaker under a pressure of 3 atmospheres in a mixture of 95 % O_2, 5 % CO_2. Thereafter tissue is fixed in 10% phosphate-buffered formalin and embedded in paraffin. Liver sections are treated with HCl for DNA denaturation and incubated with monoclonal anti-BrdU antibodies followed by an usual immunohistochemical technique. With this technique, the labelling index of replicative hepatic cells have been measured in several series of liver diseases. For instance, Shimizu et al (1988) noted that the percentage of BrdU-positive hepatocytes in hepatocarcinoma was approximately 2 fold higher in the cancerous part of the liver than in the non-cancerous part (6.4 % *versus* 3.3 %). In cirrhosis, the labelling index was low (about 2.3 %), almost equal to that observed in alcoholic liver disease (2.1%) and higher than that observed in chronic active hepatitis (0.9 %). In control subjects, the percentage of BrdU positive cells was not superior to 0.2 %, while it reached about 4% in early histological stages of primary biliary cirrhosis (Tarao et al, 1991).

Although at the present time it is too early to appreciate the significance of the values reported by Shimizu et al (1988) and Tarao et al (1991), in the diagnosis and prognosis of liver diseases, the fact that a relatively simple technique is now available to measure liver cell regeneration in human liver fragments is probably interesting. Advantages of BrdU in comparison with [^{3}H] thymidine are important : one of them is that the results can be obtained in one day only . Another is that no special equipments (dark room, etc...) is necessary.

C) DNA polymerase α

DNA polymerase α (DNA-Pα), one of the enzyme acting in DNA synthesis is present in the cell nucleus during the G1, S and G2 phases, in the cytoplasm of the cell during the M phase, but absent in the G0 phase (Seki et al, 1990). Monoclonal anti-human DNA-Pα have been prepared by Tanaka et al (1982) and have been used either *in vitro* (Bensch et al, 1982) or *in vivo* in various proliferative cells, particularly in proliferating lymphocytes (Namikawa et al, 1987).

An immunohistochemical technique is used to demonstrate DNA-Pα in the liver cells. Briefly, liver specimens obtained by needle biopsy are fixed for 6 hr in a periodate, lysine, 2% paraformaldehyde solution, then after washing in a sucrose-containing phosphate buffer frozen in liquid nitrogen (Seki et al, 1991). Cryostat sections are incubated with monoclonal antibodies which are now commercially available. An indirect immunohistochemical technique is used for the other steps. Such as for the other markers, a labelling index is measured by counting the percentage of DNA-Pα-positive cells in 1000 hepatic cells.

In a series of papers recently published, Seki et al (1990 ; 1991, a ; 1991, b) have determined with this technique the percentage of proliferating hepatic cells. In liver diseases with no proliferation, such as Gilbert disease, no DNA-Pα-positive cells was observed. Seki et al noted that proliferation was between 13 and approximately 21 % of the hepatic cells in viral hepatitis according to the clinical form of the disease (acute or fulminant hepatitis). The percentage of DNA-Pα positive-cells was higher in their patients with hepatocarcinoma (about 14 %), chronic hepatitis (5.2 %) or cirrhosis (3.8 %) that than reported by Shimizu et al (1988) in their series after BrdU incorporation. Discrepancies can be explained by the fact that DNA-Pα antibodies investigate all the phases of the cell cycle, while BrdU antibodies are limited to the S phase. In addition, patients of each series are probably different, at least with regard to liver cell regeneration, even if they presented the same histological liver disease. Whatever the explanation, DNA-Pα antibodies are at the present time the simpliest morphological method to appreciate liver cell regeneration in human liver specimens. In addition, localization of DNA-Pα can be completed by ultrastructural investigation which can be interesting to confirm light microscopic observation.

OTHERS MARKERS OF THE CELL CYCLE

[^{3}H] thymidine, BrdU and DNA-Pα do not represent all the markers of the cell cycle. Others exist but at least to our knowledge they have not been yet used in liver cell regeneration. Between the different markers, 3 nuclear proteins could be of interest : a) the proliferating cell nuclear antigen (PCNA), b) the Ki-67 nuclear antigen and c) the H3 histone mRNA.

PCNA is a nuclear protein, the auxiliary protein of another enzyme acting in DNA synthesis, the DNA polymerase δ (Bravo et al, 1987). The protein begins to be expressed in G1 phase, peaks at G1-S phase, decreases through the phase G2, and is absent in M and G0 phases (Coltrera and Gown, 1991). Monoclonal antibodies are commercially available (Garcia et al, 1989). They can be used either *in vitro* (Coltrera and Gown, 1991) or on human tissues after alcoholic fixation and paraffin embedding (Garcia et al, 1989). The Ki-67 nuclear antigen is also a nuclear antigen, expressed in S, G2 and M phases, absent in G0 phase and variably expressed in G1 phase according to the situation of the cell when entering in the cell cycle (Gerdes et al, 1984). Monoclonal antibodies are available (Coltera and Gown, 1991). The H3 histone mRNA is tightly coupled to DNA synthesis. The expression of mRNA peaks in S phase and disappears rapidly through the G2 phase ; H3 histone mRNA remains undetectable in mitotic and quiescent cells (Chou et al, 1990). No antibody is available against the H3 histone, but a cDNA has been prepared and it is possible to characterize and quantify the cell cycle phases with this probe by *in situ* hybridization.

CONCLUSION

As recalled in the introduction, the usual and simplest way to investigate liver cell regeneration by morphological methods is to search for liver cell mitoses. However, mitosis represents a small part of the cell cycle and other markers are necessary to investigate the different parts of the cycle. [³H] thymidine is the reference tool for studying the S phase. But its use needs to manipulate isotopes and the technique is time-consuming. BrdU does not present these disadvantages. Its use, based on immunocytochemistry, is within most laboratories. BrdU exploring also the S phase and providing in liver cell regeneration the same results than [³H] thymidine can be considered at the present time as the method of choice, more specially since it can be used in human liver specimens obtained by needle biopsy. The easiest method to explore liver cell regeneration in human liver specimens is to use monoclonal anti-DPNA-α antibodies. However the value of this new technique remains to be explored. In contrast to [³H] thymidine and BrdU, DNA-Pα is expressed in all the cell cycle phases except the mitotic phase and is not specific of a given phase. There are no markers capable to characterize the G1 or G2 phases only. However numerous proteins are expressed in the nucleus during the different phases of the cell cycle. Some of them are preferentially present in one or 2 phases of the cycle and could be used as markers of the cell cycle. Finally, morphological quantitative analysis can be interesting to study more precisely a given phase during liver cell regeneration.

Aknowledgments : the author wishes to thank Dr D. Bernuau and Mrs I. Tournier-Thurneyssen for providing the figures and Miss B. Le Brun for her help in the preparation of the manuscript.

REFERENCES

Bensch, K.G., Tanaka, S., Hu, S.Z., Shu-Fong, T. and Korn, D. (1982) : Intracellular localization of human DNA polymerase α with monoclonal antibodies. *J Biol Chem.* 257:8391-8396.

Barbason, H. and Van Cantfort J. (1976) : Nyctohemeral rhythms in the liver. In Progress in Liver Diseases, eds Popper H., Schaffner F., Vol V, Grune and Stratton, New York, pp 136-148.

Bravo, R., Rainer, F., Blundell, P.A. and Macdonald-Bravo, H. (1987) : Cyclin/PCNA is the auxiliary protein of DNA polymerase-δ. *Nature.* 326:515-517.

Chou, M.Y., Chang, A.L.C., McBride, J, Donoff, B., Gallagher, G.T. and Wong, D.T.W. (1990) : A rapid method to determine proliferation patterns of normal and malignant tissues by H3 mRNA by *in situ* hybridization. *Am J Pathol.* 136:729-733.

Coltrera, M.D. and Gown, A.M. (1991) : PCNA/Cyclin expression and BrdU uptake define different subpopulations in different cell lines. *J Histochem Cytochem.* 39:23-30.

Edwards, J.L. and Koch A. (1964) : Parenchymal and littoral cell proliferation during liver regeneration. Lab. Invest. 13:32-43.

Eldridge, S.R., Tilbury, L.F. Goldsworthy, T.L. and Butterworth, B.E. (1990) : Measurement of chemically induced cell proliferation in rodent liver and kidney : a comparison of 5-bromo-2'-deoxyuridine and [^{3}H] thymidine administered by injection or osmotic pump. *Carcinogenesis.* 11:2245-2251.

Fabrikant, J.I. (1968) : The kinetics of cellular proliferation in regenerating liver. *J Cell Biol.* 36:551-565.

deFazio, A., Leary, J.A., Hedley, D.W. and Tattersall, M.H.N. (1987) : Immunohistochemical detection of proliferating cells in vivo. *J Histochem Cytochem.* 35:571-577.

Frederiks, W.M., Marx, F., Chamuleau, R.A.F.M., Van Noorden, C.J.F. and James, J. (1990) : Immunocytochemical determination of ploidy class-dependent bromodeoxyuridine incorporation in rat liver parenchymal cells after partial hepatectomy. *Histochemistry.* 93:627-630.

Garcia, R.L., Coltrera, M.D. and Gown, A.M. (1989) : Analysis of proliferative grade using anti PCNA/cyclin monoclonal antibodies in fixed, embedded tissues. Comparison with flow cytometric analysis. *Am J Pathol.* 134:733-739.

Geerts, A., Lazou, J.M., De Bleser, P. and Wisse, E. (1991) : Tissue distribution, quantitation and proliferation kinetics of fat-storing cells in carbon tetrachloride-injured rat liver. *Hepatology.* 13:1193-1202.

Gerdes, J, Lemke, H, Baisch, H., Wacker, H-H., Schwabe, U and Stein, H (1984) : Cell cycle analysis of a cell proliferation-associated human nuclear antigen defined by the monoclonal antibody Ki-67. *J Immunol.* 133:1710-1715.

Gratzner, H.G. (1982) : Monoclonal antibody to 5-Bromo-and 5-Iododeoxyuridine : A new reagent for detection of DNA replication. *Science.* 218:474-475.

Gray, J.W. and Mayall, B.H. (1985) : Monoclonal antibodies against bromodeoxyuridine. Alan Riss, New York.

Grisham, J.W. (1962) : A morphologic study of deoxyribonucleic acid synthesis and cell proliferation in regenerating rat liver ; autoradiography with thymidine-H^3. *Cancer Research.* 22:842-849.

Leevy, C.M. (1963) : In vitro studies of hepatic DNA synthesis in percutaneous liver biopsy specimens. *J Lab & Clin Med.* 61:761-779.

MacDonald, R.A.(1961) : "Lifespan" of liver cells. *Arch Int Med.* 107:335-343.

Martin, E. et Feldmann, G (1983) : Histopathologie du foie et des voies biliaires. Masson, Paris.

Martin, R.L., Ilett, K.F.and Minchin, R.F. (1991).: Cell cycle-dependent uptake of putrescine and its importance in regulating cell cycle phase transition in cultured adult mouse hepatocytes. *Hepatology.* 14:1243-1250.

Namikawa, R., Ueda, R., Suchi, T. Itoh, G. Ota, K. and Takahashi, T. (1987) : Double immunoenzymatic detection of surface phenotype of proliferating lymphocytes in situ with monoclonal antibodies against DNA polymerase α and lymphocyte membrane antigens. *Am J Clin Pathol.* 87:725-731.

Paolucci, F., Mancini, R., Marucci, L., Beneditti, A., Jezequel, AM and Orlandi, F. (1990) : Immunohistochemical identification of proliferating cells following dimethylnitrosamine-induced liver injury. *Liver.* 10:278-281.

Phillips, M.J., Poucell, S. Patterson, J. and Valencia, P. (1987) : The Liver. An atlas and text of ultrastructural pathology. Raven press, New York.

Rabes, H.M. (1976) : Kinetics of hepatocellular proliferation after partial resection of the liver. In Progress in Liver Diseases. eds Popper H., Schaffner F. Vol. V, Grune and Stratton, New York. pp 83-99

Sand, T.E., Gladhaug, I.P., Refsnes, M. and Christoffersen, T. (1989).: DNA synthesis in cultured adult rat hepatocytes : effect of serum and calcium. *Liver.* 9:20-26.

Schutte, B., Reynders, M.M.J., Bosman, F.T. and Blijham, G.H. (1987) : Effect of tissue fixation on anti-bromodeoxyuridine immunohistochemistry. *J Histochem Cytochem.* 35:1343-1345.

Seki, S., Sakaguchi, H., Kawakita, N., Yanai, A., Kim, K., Mizoguchi, Y. and Kobayashi, K. (1990) : Identification and fine structure of proliferating hepatocytes in malignant and nonmalignant liver diseases by use of a monoclonal antibody against DNA polymerase alpha. *Hum Pathol.* 21:1020-1030.

Seki, S., Sakaguchi, H., Kawakita, N. Yanai, A., Kuroki, T., Mizoguchi, Y., Kobayashi, K. and Monna, T. (1991, a) : Detection of proliferating hepatocytes in patients with acute hepatic failure by mitotic figures and a monoclonal antibody against DNA polymerase alpha.*Liver.* 11:118-126.

Seki, S., Sakaguchi, H., Kawakita, N., Yanai, A., Kuroki, T., Mizoguchi, Y., Kobayashi, K. and Monna, T. (1991, b) : Detection of proliferating liver cells in various diseases by a monoclonal antibody against DNA polymerase-α : with special reference to the relationship between hepatocytes and sinusoidal cells. *Hepatology.* 14:781-788.

Shimizu, A., Tarao, K. Takemiya, S; Harada, M., Inoue, T. and Ono, T. (1988) : S-phase cells in diseased human liver determined by an *in vitro* BrdU-anti-BrdU method. *Hepatology.* 8:1535-1539.

Tanaka, S., Hu, S.-Z., Wang, T.S.F., and Korn, D. (1982) : Preparation and preliminary characterization of monoclonal antibodies against DNA polymerase α. *J Biol Chem*, 257:8386-8390.

Tanaka, Y. Mak, K.M. and Lieber, C.S. (1990) : Immunohistochemical detection of proliferating lipocytes in regenerating rat liver. *J Pathol.* 160:129-134.

Tarao, K, Shimizu, A. Ohkawa, S. Harada, M., Ito, Y. Tamai, S., Kuni, Y., Nagaoka, T. and Hoshino, H. (1991) : Increased uptake of bromodeoxyuridine by hepatocytes from early stage of primary biliary cirrhosis. *Gastroenterology.* 100:725-730.

Tomomura, A., Sawada, N., Sattler, G.L., Kleinman, H.K. and Pitot, H.C.(1987) : The control of DNA synthesis in primary cultures of hepatocytes from adult and young rats : interactions of extracellular matrix components, epidermal growth factor, and the cell cycle *J Cell Physiol.* 130:221-227.

Liver stem cells : myth or reality ?

Jean-Yves Scoazec

Laboratoire de Biologie Cellulaire and INSERM U.327, Faculté de Médecine Xavier Bichat, 16 rue Henri Huchard, 75018 Paris, France

The search for liver stem cells is a long-standing quest in hepatology. The answer to this issue is not only important for the understanding of experimental liver regeneration, but becomes of increasing relevance for the correct evaluation of many aspects of human liver pathology, including the mechanisms of liver cell regeneration after severe injury, the patterns of bile duct proliferation, and the initial phases of liver carcinogenesis.

We will successively review the following points : (a) the stem cell concept, (b) the role of stem cells in liver organogenesis, and (c) the arguments supporting the existence of stem cells in the adult liver and their possible role in normal and pathologic liver.

THE STEM CELL CONCEPT

It is usually assumed that all the mature cells of an adult tissue, even when they belong to several lineages differing in structure and/in function, derive from the multiplication and differentiation of a unique stem cell. This process is particularly obvious during embryogenesis and organogenesis in which each step of differentiation is represented by pure populations. The same process persists in adult life, to allow the permanent renewal of mature cells lost after their normal life span or the restoration of organ integrity after injury.

Most of the current concepts about the role and regulation of stem cell differentiation derive from the study of hematopoiesis and, particularly, of myelopoiesis. All circulating myeloid cells, representing four distinct lineages (erythrocytic, granulo-monocytic, eosinophilic and megakaryocytic), derive from a common myeloid stem cell, located within the bone marrow (Quesenberry and Levitt, 1979; Clark & Kamen, 1987; Sieff, 1987). Myelopoiesis involves three successive steps : (a) pluripotent myeloid stem cells common to all myeloid lineages differentiate from totipotent stem cells common to both lymphoid and myeloid lineages, (b) pluripotent stem cells differentiate into several types of progenitor cells: each progenitor cell is committed to a distinct myeloid lineage, and (c) progenitor cells, stimulated by the appropriate growth factors, engage into a phase of clonal expansion coupled with progressive differentiation; the two processes are parallel but inversely correlated: schematically, the more differentiated the cell is, the less proliferative it is.

Many tissues are organized according to the same model (Marceau, 1990). Most adult epithelia, including epidermis, transitional, gastric and intestinal epithelia, contain three identifiable compartments: (a) a stem cell compartment, including totipotent and pluripotent stem cells, capable of auto-replication, and not engaged into a process of differentiation, (b) a compartment of committed or progenitor cells, irreversibly engaged along one line of differentiation, and (c) a compartment of differentiating cells (Fig. 1). This organization allows the permanent renewal of mature cells lost after their normal life span. However, some adult tissues do not fit this model. Muscular and nervous tissues do not contain stem cells and their differentiated cells are not replaced. What is the situation in the liver? Is the liver organized like most other epithelia or, in contrast, like some non-epithelial tissues?

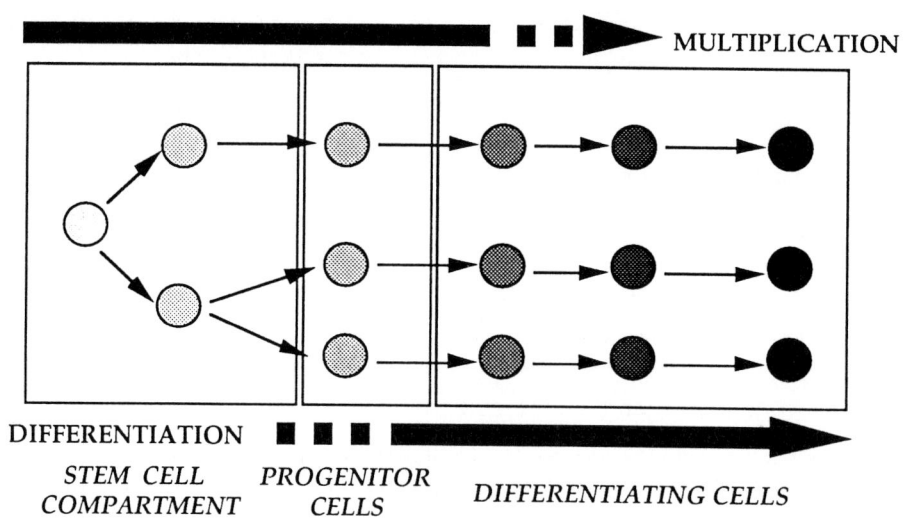

Fig. 1. Role of stem cells in organogenesis and cell renewal

To address these issues, we will successively examine two questions : (a) the role of stem cells in liver organogenesis, (b) the arguments supporting the existence of stem cells in adult normal liver.

ROLE OF STEM CELLS IN NORMAL LIVER ORGANOGENESIS

Adult liver contains two distinct epithelial lineages : hepatocytes and bile duct cells. Pluripotent stem cells common to both hepatocytes and bile duct cells have been identified during rat liver embryogenesis (Shiojiri, 1984; van Eyken *et al.*, 1988; Marceau, 1990). Such stem cells, or hepatoblasts, give rise to two distinct types of progenitor cells, one for the hepatocytic lineage, and one for the bile duct lineage (Fig. 2). In the rat, the two lineages are fully separated at the fifteenth embryonic day. The steps involved in the progressive differentiation of progenitor cells into mature hepatocytes and bile duct cells are not yet fully characterized. Certain indirect arguments suggest that the liver pluripo-

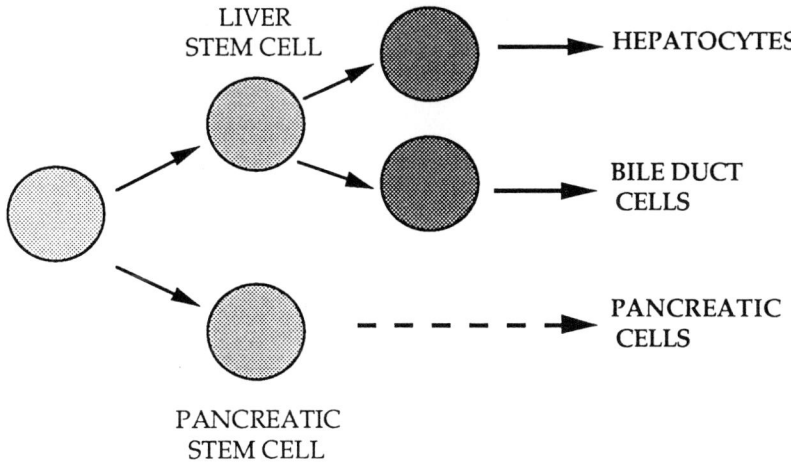

Fig. 2. Role of stem cells in liver organogenesis

tent stem cell itself derives from a totipotent stem cell common to both hepatic and pancreatic cells. It is actually possible to induce the differentiation of pancreatic ductal cells into fully mature hepatocytes in rats fed a copper-deficient diet containing a metal chelator (Rao *et al.*, 1989).

PRESENCE AND ROLE OF STEM CELLS IN THE NORMAL ADULT LIVER

The presence of stem cells in the normal adult liver has long been contested for several reasons :

(a) hepatocytes have a long life span, estimated to 200 to 400 days, and their physiological renewal is exceedingly low (Leffert *et al.*, 1988; Fausto, 1990);

(b) in contrast to most other mature, differentiated epithelial cells, hepatocytes retain a replicative capacity : they are able to multiplicate in response to growth stimuli (Leffert *et al.*, 1988; Fausto, 1990);

(c) the auto-replicative capacity of normal adult hepatocytes is sufficient to allow the complete restoration of the liver mass after surgical hepatectomy (Leffert *et al.*, 1988; Fausto & Mead, 1989; Fausto, 1990) : therefore, it is likely that this capacity is sufficient to ensure the physiological renewal of hepatocytes in the normal situation.

However, several arguments concur to suggest the presence of a stem cell compartment in the adult liver. The three main arguments to support this concept are : (a) the streaming liver theory, (b) the mechanisms of bile duct cell renewal, and (c) the emergence of new epithelial populations after severe hepatocyte agression. Let us successively examine those three points.

The streaming liver theory

The streaming liver theory postulates that hepatocyte renewal is vectorial along the liver lobule (Zajicek *et al.*, 1985; Arber *et al.*, 1988). Newly formed hepatocytes would appear into the periportal region of the lobule, then migrate along the trabeculae at a nearly constant speed, and finally disappear in the perivenous region of the lobule, at the end of their normal life span. This is in accordance with the fact that periportal hepatocytes are the main proliferative cells after partial hepatectomy. These observations would therefore suggest the existence of a compartment of hepatocyte progenitors in the periportal area. While this theory had gained a large accceptance, the experimental data on which it is founded have been recently discussed. New experiments actually suggest that hepatocyte renewal is not vectorial within the hepatic lobule, but might occur in any point of the liver parenchyma (Slott *et al.*, 1990; Schuler *et al.*, 1991). Further studies are necessary to clarify this issue.

The mechanisms of bile duct cell renewal

The mechanisms of bile duct cell renewal are not well known (Arber & Zajicek, 1990; Slott *et al.*, 1990; Zajicek, 1991). By analogy with other simple digestive epithelia, such as those of stomach or intestine, it might be expected that bile duct epithelium contains a stem cell compartment, ensuring the permanent renewal of mature bile duct cells after their normal life span. This is not in contradiction with the fact that, like hepatocytes, mature bile duct cells seem to retain replicative capacities (Slott *et al.*, 1990). This situation is known in other epithelia : for instance, the renewal of the urinary transitional epithelium is ensured both by the replication of mature, differentiated transitional cells and by the continuous process of differentiation of resident stem cells (Marceau, 1990).

Certain observations performed in human pathology suggest the existence of bile duct cell progenitors in adult liver. It has been shown that proliferating bile duct cells appearing in long-standing cholestasis express the neural cell adhesion molecule (Roskams *et al.*, 1990). This cell adhesion molecule, absent from adult epithelial cells, is transiently expressed by embryonic epithelial cells during their normal process of differentiation. The expression of this molecule by proliferating bile duct cells in pathological situations might therefore indicate the commitment of biliary progenitors in the formation of new bile ducts.

The emergence of new epithelial cell populations after severe toxic injury of the liver : the case of oval cells

Oval cells are epithelial cells which rapidly proliferate in rat liver after carcinogen treatment and chemically induced severe liver injury. Oval cells are small, rounded cells, with a high nucleo-cytoplasmic ratio, which first appear in periportal areas and rapidly expand through the hepatic parenchyma (Farber, 1956). They constitute a highly pleiomorphic population (Marceau, 1990; Sirica *et al.*, 1990), which has long been suspected to result from the proliferation of liver stem cells. Two distinct questions are therefore raised : (a) do oval cells behave as hepatic stem cells ?, (b) in this case, are they in some help to identify stem cells in normal adult liver ? Let us successively examine those two points.

To consider that oval cells behave as stem cells, they must fulfill the following three criteria : (a) they must be highly replicative cells, (b) certain oval cells must look like fetal hepatoblasts, and (c) oval cells must be able to differentiate along both biliary and hepatocytic lineages. It is well established that oval cells are highly replicative cells with a short life span. They are able to incorporate high levels of tritiated thymidine : after carcinogen administration, they contain the highest levels of tritiated thymidine amongst all the liver cell populations (Sell, 1990). Furthermore, oval cells exhibit high levels of expression of oncogenes known to be associated with the cell cycle, such as c-*myc*, c-*fos* and c-*ras* (Yaswen *et al.*, 1985; Braun *et al.*, 1989). Oval cell proliferation remains regulated : for instance, oval cells expressed high levels of the p53 protein, a so-called anti-oncogene controlling the entry in the cell cycle (Braun *et al*, 1989).

A further argument to consider oval cells as representative of presumptive stem cells is that certain oval cells actually resemble hepatoblasts. Like hepatoblasts, most oval cells coexpress high levels of α-fetoprotein (AFP) and moderate levels of albumin (Petropoulos *et al.*, 1985; Germain *et al.*, 1988a; Scoazec *et al.*, 1989). Oval cells contain the 2.3-kilobase AFP mRNA characteristic of fetal hepatocytes and absent from adult hepatocytes (Petropoulos *et al.*, 1985). Finally, certain oval cells coexpress surface markers respectively considered as specific for mature bile duct cells and for mature hepatocytes (Marceau, 1990; Sirica *et al.*, 1990).

What are the capacities of differentiation of oval cells ? It must be first pointed out that the majority of oval cells disappears by apoptosis and does not differentiate (Sirica *et al.*, 1990). Most of the remaining population differentiate into cells of biliary lineage : this point has been well established, both *in vivo* and *in vitro*, on morphological, biochemical and phenotypical grounds (Germain *et al.*, 1985; Bannasch & Zerban, 1986; Germain *et al.*, 1988a; Germain *et al.*, 1988b; Sirica *et al.*, 1990). The most controversial issue is to assess whether oval cells are able to differentiate into cells of hepatocytic lineage. The first evidence presented to support this concept is the identification of cells considered as intermediate between oval cells and hepatocytes in certain models of chemical hepatocarcinogenesis (Farber, 1956; Inaoka, 1967; Iwasaki *et al.*, 1972; Guillouzo *et al.*, 1978; Sell, 1980; Guillouzo *et al.*, 1981). These so-called transitional cells look like small, rounded hepatocytes, express both AFP and albumin, contain the same fetal isoenzymes than oval cells and display a complex admixture of surface markers characteristic either for oval cells or for hepatocytes. Such observations have prompted *in vitro* and *in vivo* experiments aimed to evaluate the capacities of hepatocytic differentiation of oval cells. *In vitro*, it is possible to force oval cells isolated from the livers of carcinogen-treated rats to differentiate into cells presenting certain hepatocytic features, such as the capacity for albumin synthesis (Germain *et al.*, 1988a; Germain *et al.*, 1988b). However, such induced cells never present the whole spectrum of terminal hepatocytic differentiation. *In vivo*, the bulk of evidence is greater. Despite initial contradictory results (Grisham et Porta, 1964; Sell *et al.*, 1981; Tatematsu *et al.*, 1984), it has been more recently convincingly demonstrated that, in certain models of chemical hepatocarcinogenesis, oval cells might transform into cells with an hepatocytic phenotype (Evarts *et al.*, 1987; Evarts *et al.*, 1989). The intermediate stages of this differentiation process have been partly characterized (Evarts *et al.*, 1989; Evarts *et al.*, 1990). However, the products of oval cell differentiation are not mature normal hepatocytes. They correspond to the so-called basophilic hepatocytes, a cell population specific for the carcinogen-induced hyperplastic nodules observed at the early stages of chemical hepatocarcinogenesis. Like oval cells, basophilic hepatocytes have a short life span, highly replicative capacities and coexpress AFP and albumin (Evarts *et al.*, 1989; Scoazec *et al.*, 1989). They have often been considered as the immediate precursors of malignant cells (Farber, 1976). In summary, good experimental evidence shows that oval cells might differentiate into cells of bile duct lineage. However, while some oval cells might evolve into cells displaying a few hepatocytic features, there is no definitive argument showing that oval cells are able to form fully differentiated hepatocytes. Further studies are necessary to assess whether or not oval cells actually behave as hepatocyte progenitors and what are the growth and differentiation factors needed to overcome the apparent block of differentiation observed in most *in vivo* and *in vitro* situations.

Despite these limitations, do oval cells help to identify stem cells in the normal adult liver ? In other terms, is it possible to use the characteristic features of oval cells as probes to search for presumptive stem cells in the normal hepatic tissue ? Certain "non parenchymal epithelial cells" isolated from normal rat livers actually exhibit some of the characteristics of oval cells : (a) expression of oval cell surface markers (Marceau, 1990), (b) expression of the same profile of enzyme markers (Tsao *et al.*, 1984), (c) expression of the 2.3-kilobase AFP mRNA found in fetal liver cells and oval cells (Petropoulos *et al.*, 1985). It is therefore possible that the existence of such cells indicates the presence of a stem cell compartment in the normal liver.

The last question to address is to determine the location of the presumptive liver stem cells in the normal adult liver. It is usually assumed that presumptive hepatic stem cells are located within the cholangiolar wall (Sell, 1990; Marceau, 1990). Cholangioles, or bile ductules, are short segments of the biliary tree, located in the immediate periportal region (Schaffner et Popper, 1961). They are directly connected with bile canaliculi and precede the first interlobular bile ducts. Arguments supporting the location of stem cells in the cholangiolar wall are of different types : (a) the initial site of oval cell or ductular proliferation in the injured liver is always periportal, (b) the first cells to incorporate tritiated thymidine after liver injury are small epithelial cells located in the periportal zone (Sell et Salman, 1984), (c) the few adult epithelial liver cells to retain the fetal-type of AFP mRNA are situated in the same region (Lemire et Fausto, 1991). However, at ultrastructural examination, cholangiolar cells always appear as well-differentiated simple epithelial cells and display none of the morphological features expected to characterize presumptive stem cells (Tavoloni, 1987; Sirica *et al.*, 1990). Nevertheless, this does not exclude the presence of scattered stem cells within cholangioles. Stem cells, even where they are comparatively abundant, such as in myeloid tissue, are always morphologically elusive.

CONCLUSION

The following conclusions might be proposed regarding the existence and role of stem cells in the normal adult liver. It is likely that adult liver contains a stem cell compartment, consisting of pluripotent stem cells, bile duct cell progenitors and hepatocyte progenitors. In the normal state, liver stem cells do not participate in the renewal of mature hepatocytes, which retain sufficient auto-replicative capacities to maintain their normal numbers. The participation of this presumptive stem cell compartment to bile duct cell renewal has yet to be evaluated. In situations of regeneration without injury, the auto-replicative capacities of mature hepatocytes are sufficient to restore liver integrity without commitment of the stem cell compartment. In situations of regeneration with injury or in the case of experimental chemical hepatocarcinogenesis, when the auto-replicative capacities of mature liver epithelial cells are superated or inhibited, the proliferation and differentiation of liver stem cells are stimulated. Liver stem cells might therefore be considered as "facultative" stem cells (Grisham, 1980). However, most of the patterns and steps of their process of differentiation have yet to be determined.

REFERENCES

Arber, N. & Zajicek, G. (1990): The streaming liver. IV. Streaming intrahepatic bile ducts. *Liver* 10, 137-140.

Arber, N., Zajicek, G. *et al* (1988) The streaming liver. II. Hepatocyte life history. *Liver* 8, 80-87.

Bannasch, P. & Zerban, H. (1986): Pathogenesis of primary liver tumors induced by chemicals. *Rec. Results Cancer Res.* 100, 1-15.

Braun, L., Mikumo, R. *et al* (1989): Production of hepatocellular carcinoma by oval cells : cell cycle expression of *c-myc* and p53 at different stages of oval cell transformation. *Cancer Res.* 49, 1554-1561.

Clark, S.C. & Kamen, T. (1987): The human hematopoietic colony-stimulating factors. *Science* 236, 1229-1237.

Evarts, R.P., Nagy, P. *et al* (1987): A precursor-product relationship between oval cells and hepatocytes in rat liver. *Carcinogenesis* 8, 1737-1740.

Evarts, R.P., Nagy, P. *et al* (1989): *In vivo* differentiation of rat liver oval cells into hepatocytes. *Cancer Res.* 49, 1541-1546.

Evarts, R.P., Nakatsukasa, H. *et al* (1990): Cellular and molecular changes in the early stages of chemical hepatocarcinogenesis in the rat. *Cancer Res.* 50, 3439-3444.

Farber, E. (1956): Similarities in the sequence of early histological changes induced in the liver of the rat by ethionine, 2-acetylaminofluorene, and 3'-methyl-4-dimethylaminoazobenzene. *Cancer Res.* 16, 142-155.

Farber, E. (1976): Hyperplastic areas, hyperplastic nodules, and hyperbasophilic areas as putative precursor lesions. *Cancer Res.* 36, 2532-2533.

Fausto, N. & Mead, J.E. (1989): Regulation of liver growth: protooncogenes and transforming growth factors. *Lab. Invest.* 60, 4-13.

Fausto, N. (1990): Hepatocyte differentiation and liver progenitor cells. *Curr. Opin. Cell Biol.* 2, 1036-1042.

Germain, L., Blouin, M.J. et al (1988a): Biliary epithelial and hepatocytic cell lineage relationships in embryonic rat liver as determined by the differential expression of cytokeratins, α-fetoprotein, albumin and cell surface-exposed components. *Cancer Res.* 48, 4909-4918.

Germain, L., Goyette, R. et al (1985): Differential cytokeratin and α-fetoprotein expression in morphologically distinct epithelial cells emerging at the early stage of rat hepatocarcinogenesis. *Cancer Res.* 45, 673-681.

Germain, L., Noel, M. et al (1988b) Promotion of growth and differentiation of rat ductular oval cells in primary culture. *Cancer Res.* 48, 368-378.

Grisham, J.W. & Porta, E.A. (1964): Origin and fate of proliferated hepatic ductal cells: electronmicroscopic and autoradiographic studies. *Exp. Mol. Pathol.* 2, 242-261.

Grisham, J.W. (1980): Cell types in long-term propagable cultures of rat liver. *Ann. N. Y. Acad. Sci.* 349, 128-137.

Guillouzo, A., Belanger, L. et al (1978): Cellular and subcellular immunolocalization of α_1-fetoprotein and albumin in rat liver. Reevaluation of various experimental conditions. *J. Histochem. Cytochem.* 26, 948-959.

Guillouzo, A., Weber, A. et al (1981): Cell types involved in the expression of foetal aldolases during rat azo-dye hepatocarcinogenesis. *J. Cell Sci.* 49, 249-260.

Inaoka, Y. (1967): Significance of the so-called oval cell proliferation during azo-dye hepatocarcinogenesis. *Gann* 58, 355-366.

Iwasaki, T., Dempo, K. et al (1972): Fluctuation of various cell populations and their characteristics during azo-dye carcinogenesis. *Gann* 63, 21-30.

Leffert, H.L., Koch, K.S. et al (1988): Hepatocyte regeneration, replication, and differentiation. In *The Liver : Biology and Pathobiology*, ed. Arias, I.M., Jakoby, W.B., Popper, H., Schachter, D. & Shafritz, D.A., pp 1125-1146. New York:Raven Press.

Lemire, J.M. & Fausto, N. (1991): Multiple α-fetoprotein RNAs in adult rat liver. Cell-type specific expression and differential regulation. *Cancer Res.* 51, 4656-4664.

Marceau, N. (1990): Cell lineages and differentiation programs in epidermal, urothelial and hepatic tissues and their neoplasms. *Lab. Invest.* 63, 4-20.

Petropoulos, C.J., Yaswen, P. et al (1985): Cell lineages in liver carcinogenesis: possible clues from studies of the distribution of α-fetoprotein RNA sequences in cell populations isolated from normal, regenerating, and preneoplastic rat livers. *Cancer Res.* 45, 5762-5768.

Quesenberry, P. & Levitt, L. (1979): Hematopoietic stem cells. *New Engl. J. Med.* 301, 755-760, 819-823, 868-872.

Rao, M.S., Dwivedi, R.S. et al (1989): Role of periductal and ductular epithelial cells of the adult rat pancreas in pancreatic hepatocyte lineage. *Am. J. Pathol.* 134, 1069-1086.

Roskams, T., van den Oord, J.J. et al (1990): Neuroendocrine features of reactive bile ductules in cholestatic liver disease. *Am. J. Pathol.* 137, 1019-1025.

Schaffner, F. & Popper, H. (1961): Electron microscopic studies of normal and proliferated bile ductules. *Am. J. Pathol.* 38, 393-410.

Schuler, E., Salvi, R. et al (1991): Pattern of hepatocyte renewal in regenerated rat liver. Evidence against a streaming mechanism (abstract). *Hepatology* 14, 102A.

Scoazec, J.-Y., Moreau, A. et al (1989): Cellular expression of α-fetoprotein gene and its relation to albumin gene expression during rat azo-dye hepatocarcinogenesis. *Cancer Res.* 49, 1790-1796.

Sell, S. & Salman, J. (1984): Light and electron microscopic autoradiographic analysis of proliferating cells during the early stages of chemical hepatocarcinogenesis in the rat induced by feeding N-2-fluorenylacetamide in a choline deficient diet. *Am. J. Pathol.* 114, 287-300.

Sell, S. (1980): Heterogeneity of alpha-fetoprotein (AFP) and albumin containing cells in normal and pathological permissive states for AFP production : AFP containing cells induced in adult rats recapitulate the appearance of AFP containing hepatocytes in fetal rats. *Oncodev. Biol. Med.* 1, 93-105.

Sell, S. (1990): Is there a liver stem cell? *Cancer Res.* 50, 3811-3815.

Sell, S., Osborn, R. et al (1981): Autoradiography of "oval cells" appearing rapidly in the livers of rats fed N-2-fluorenylacetamide in a choline deficient diet. *Carcinogenesis* 2, 7-14.

Shiojiri, N. (1984): The origin of intrahepatic bile duct cells in the mouse. *J. Embryol. Exp. Morph.* 79, 25-39.

Sieff, C.A. (1987): Hematopoietic growth factors. *J. Clin. Invest.* 79, 1549-1557.

Sirica, A.E., Mathis, G.A. et al (1990): Isolation, culture, and transplantation of intrahepatic biliary epithelial cells and oval cells. *Pathobiology* 58, 44-64.

Slott, P.A., Liu, M.H. et al (1990): Origin, pattern, and mechanism of bile duct proliferation following biliary obstruction in the rat. *Gastroenterology* 99, 466-477.

Tatematsu, M., Ho, R.H. et al (1984): Studies on proliferation and fate of oval cells in the liver of rats treated with 2-acetyl-aminofluorene and partial hepatectomy. *Am. J. Pathol.* 114, 418-430.

Tavoloni, N. (1987): The intrahepatic biliary epithelium : an area of growing interest in hepatology. *Semin. Liver. Dis.* 7, 280-292.

Tsao, M.S., Smith, J.D. et al (1984): A diploid epithelial cell line from normal adult rat liver with phenotypic properties of "oval" cells. *Exp. Cell. Res.* 154, 38-52.

van Eyken, P., Sciot, R. et al (1988): Intrahepatic bile duct development in the rat : a cytokeratin immunohistochemical study. *Lab. Invest.* 59, 52-59.

Yaswen, P., Goyette, M. *et al* (1985): Expression of c-Ki-*ras*, c-Ha-*ras*, and c-*myc* in specific cell types during hepatocarcinogenesis. *Mol. Cell. Biol.* 5, 780-786.

Zajicek, G. (1991): Hepatocytes and intrahepatic bile duct epithelium originate from a common stem cell. *Gastroenterology* 100, 582-583.

Zajicek, G., Oren, R. *et al* (1985): The streaming liver. *Liver* 5, 293-300.

Role of sinusoidal cells in liver regeneration

Paulette Bioulac-Sage, Liliane Dubuisson, Brigitte Le Bail, Pierre Bernard, Jacques Carles, Patrick Lefebvre, Charles Balabaud

Laboratoire des Interactions Cellulaires, Université de Bordeaux II, Laboratoire d'Anatomie Pathologique et Unité de Transplantation Hépatique, Hôpital Pellegrin, Service des Maladies de l'Appareil Digestif et de Chirurgie digestive, Hôpital Saint-André, CHRU Bordeaux, France

INTRODUCTION

The specificity of the highly efficient vascularization system of the liver (25% of total blood output transits through the liver) lies in its dual blood supply and in the special type of capillary which forms the irrigation network. Arterial blood supplies 20% of the total hepatic blood flow. Portal blood (80% of total hepatic blood flow) contains blood from the pancreas, the digestive tract, the spleen and the biliary tree and is enriched with nutrients and hormones.

The hepatocyte by its 2 sinusoidal poles, is in contact through the Disse space with a unique capillary, the sinusoid, which itself is limited by a thin fenestrated endothelial barrier. Anchored to this barrier, the Kupffer cell (KC) is a resident macrophage. Liver-associated lymphocytes (LAL) which are in contact with the KC and/or the endothelial cell (EC) contain a high % of NK cells (33%). Delimited by the sinusoidal membrane of the hepatocyte covered by microvilli and by the abluminal membrane of the EC, the Disse space contains a specific extracellular matrix (ECM) with no real basement membrane (BM) and perisinusoidal cells (PSC) with cell bodies often rich in lipid droplets containing vitamin A and thin, discontinuous processes which surround the endothelial barrier.

Although more attention has been focussed on hepatocytes, it has been largely documented that cell/cell (hepatocytes/non-parenchymal cells) and cell/matrix interactions are of prime importance for liver homeostasis in spite of the fact that non-parenchymal cells represent only a small fraction of the liver parenchyma (Blouin *et al.*,1977) (Table 1- Fig.1); it is thus impossible to conceive liver regeneration *in vivo* as being simply a question of hepatocytes. If we take the most frequently used model of regeneration, partial hepatectomy (PH), we find that, one week after surgery, the liver has almost recovered its preoperative weight and liver architecture is grossly normal (Fausto,1990). The proliferation of hepatocytes has been accompagnied by the formation of new sinusoids (Martinez-Hernandez *et al.*,1991).

There are several arguments to suggest that sinusoidal cells play a role in liver regeneration, particularly: 1) the cytolocalization of growth factors in sinusoidal cells and 2) morphological evidence of mitosis and ultrastructural changes in sinusoidal cells occurring during regeneration.

Methods for studying the role of sinusoidal cells in liver regeneration encounter two main difficulties: 1) accurate identification *in vivo* of the type of sinusoidal cells involved is extremely difficult without using ultrastructural techniques with perfusion-fixed material, 2) it is virtually impossible, at least with human liver, to obtain *in vitro* a reasonably pure population of sinusoidal cells.

TABLE 1. SINUSOIDS - MORPHOMETRY [1]
Sinusoidal volume : 15.5%
  - lumen : 10.6%
  - Disse space : 4.9%

Sinusoidal cells :
  - 6.3% of liver parenchyma
    . EC : 2.8%
    . KC : 2.1%
    . PSC : 1.4%
  - 26.5% of liver plasma membranes
    . large plasma membrane surface of EC and PSC+++
    . importance of lysosomal volume in KC and EC

[1] Adult rat liver (Blouin *et al.*, 1977)

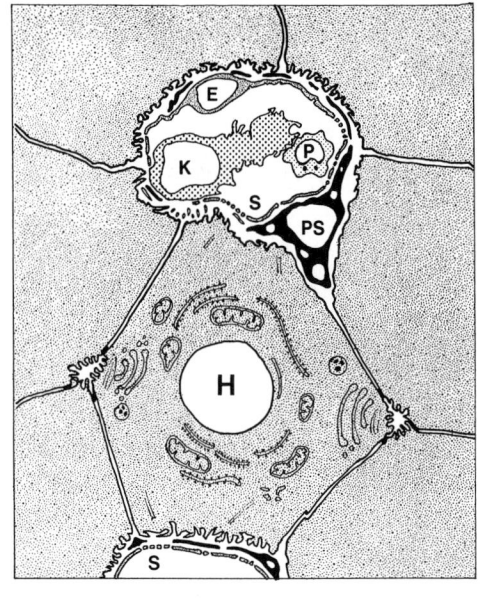

Fig.1. Schematic representation of a sinusoid (S) surrounded by several hepatocytes (H); K: Kupffer cell; E: endothelial cell; PS: perisinusoidal cell; P: pit cell (liver large granular lymphocyte)

Table 2. HEPATIC REGENERATION : MODELS
1 - *Partial hepatectomy* (50-90%- usually [rat] 75%)
2 - *Necrosis*
.acute(subfulminant, fulminant hepatic failure)[1]
.chronic (cirrhosis - regenerative nodules)[2]
3 - *Vascular disorders*
. FNH: tumor (hyperarterialization)[3]
. NRH: nodular hypertrophy (well-vascularized zones) contrasting with atrophy (poorly-vascularized zones)[4]
4 - *Clonal proliferation of hepatocytes*
. adenoma (benign)[3,5]
. hepatocellular carcinoma (malignant)[3,6]

FNH : focal nodular hyperplasia; NRH : nodular regenerative hyperplasia [1]Kawakika *et al.*, 1991 [2]Callea *et al.*, 1991; Bioulac-Sage *et al.*, 1992b [3]Bioulac-Sage *et al.*, 1988 [4]Bioulac-Sage *et al.*, 1992a [5]Bioulac-Sage *et al.*, 1986 [6]Tabarin *et al.*, 1986; Seki *et al.*, 1991

It has also been shown that mechanisms operating *in vitro* may not operate *in vivo* as shown recently in the dog with the Eck fistula model (Francavilla *et al.*, 1991).
The aim of this study is to summarize the few data we already have on the cytolocalization of growth factors in sinusoidal cells and on the morphology of these cells. Although the most widely used model for the study of liver regeneration is PH, we have also included data obtained from other models (Table 2).

I - LOCALIZATION OF HEPATOCYTE GROWTH FACTORS IN NON-PARENCHYMAL CELLS

Localization *in vitro* of the major peptide growth factors which induce mitogenic activity in hepatocytes reveals the wide distribution of these factors (Table 3). Concerning the liver, it is of interest to note that in normal conditions HGF is absent in hepatocytes in both the rat and humans but present in the biliary, vascular EC, KC and PSC of the rat, and biliary and vascular EC in humans (Wolf *et al.*, 1991; Schirmacher *et al.*, 1992; Michalopoulos & Zarnegar, 1992). Expression of HGF increases after CCl4 injury but not (or less) after PH (Noji *et al.*, 1990). The localization of TGF β is very similar to that of HGF apart from the fact that KC are not labelled, whereas PSC and cells around portal veins are. The latter may possibly be stem cells. Expression increases after PH (Nakatsukasa *et al.*, 1990).

Table 3. HEPATOCYTE GROWTH FACTORS
a) PEPTIDE GROWTH FACTORS : HEPATOCYTE MITOGENS (main source) [1]

TGF α : fibroblasts, embryonic cells, brain tissue, keratinocytes, monocytes, carcinoma
EGF: gastrointestinal glands - a FGF : endothelial cells - IGF-II : liver (sinusoidal cells) [2]
HSS : hepatocytes - HGF: widely distributed (epithelial cells..., liver : EC, KC)
HSS: Hepatocyte stimulating substance [1]Andus *et al.*,1991; [2]Zindy *et al.*,1992

b) LOCALIZATION OF HEPATOCYTE GROWTH FACTOR (HGF) IN HUMAN AND RAT LIVER

	H	Biliary C intra	Biliary C extra	EC PV	EC CV	EC SEC	KC	PSC
Rat	-[1]	-	+	+	+	-[+][2]	+[+]	+[3]
Human	-	+	+	+	+	-	-	

. under normal condition : [1] *immunohistochemistry* (polyclonal antiserum to HGF) - Wolf *et al.*, 1991 ; [2] *in situ hybridization* - Noji *et al.*,1990. [3] *in situ hybridization* - Schirmacher *et al.*, 1992
. after injury (CCl4)[2]: increased expression - after PH[2]: no (or less) change

c) LOCALIZATION OF TGF B IN THE LIVER (*hybridization in situ, immunohistochemistry*) *

	H	Periductal cell	PV	CV	PSC	Capsule	EC
Control (rat liver)	-	+	++[1]	++	+	+	+[2]
PH	-	+++	+++ (early peak 12-24h)				+[3]

[1] around (stem cells ?) [2] some sinusoidal EC (SEC) [3] EC of blood vessels
* Nakatsukasa *et al.*,1990

II- MORPHOLOGY OF NON-PARENCHYMAL CELLS AND OF THE ECM DURING PH

Mitosis of sinusoidal cells is delayed, in comparison with that of hepatocytes ((Widmann & Fahimi, 1976, Martinez-Hernandez *et al.*, 1991, Tanaka *et al.*,1991) ; this leads initially to the formation of clusters of hepatocytes and the widening of hepatic plates. During regeneration, sinusoidal cells are in a state of activation. Major ultrastructural findings are summarized in Table 4 and Fig. 2-3. As shown, very little data has been published on EC and PSC.Two and four days after PH, PSC have the morphological characteristics of fibroblasts with a very active RER, whilst EC are involved in a dynamic process that evokes angiogenesis (see below). As a result of PH there is initially an increase in cell mass with no concomitant increase in ECM which leads to a decrease in the ECM/cell mass ratio. This ratio returns to normal when regeneration is completed. Of the ECM components, laminin is the one that shows the most dramatic changes with prominent intracellular staining of PSC and a maximum staining of the Disse space at 48 hours. It is of interest to note that there is no deposit of basement membrane. The marked expression of laminin and the fact that it could exercise a function in morphogenesis would suggest that it may play a critical role in the reorganization of the regenerating liver (Table 5) (Martinez-Hernandez *et al.*,1991).

Table 4. LIVER REGENERATION - PARTIAL HEPATECTOMY -

MORPHOLOGY OF LGL, KC [1]
Increase in the number of LGL and KC after PH
 - peak (7-14 days). KC x 2 ; LGL x 3
 - mitosis: frequent between 1-5 days (KC : peak at 2 days), rare after 7 days (cells of extrahepatic origin)
 - numerous, close and wide-surfaced contacts between KC and LGL

Signs of morphological activation
 - KC: numerous cytoplasmic projections, many vacuoles and phagolysosomes, occasional worm-like structures, numerous vesicles at the areas of contact KC / LGL
 - LGL: some cells in the Disse space, numerous granules and rod-cored vesicles (no quantitative data) * increase antitumor response after PH[2]

MORPHOLOGY OF SINUSOIDAL ENDOTHELIAL CELLS [3,4,*]
Mitotic index: slow increase with a peak at 4 days (delay compared to KC)
Morphology
 - elongated shape, many micropinocytotic vesicles and a few larger cytoplasmic vacuoles
 - a fairly straight luminal plasma membrane with focal fenestration
 - cytoplasm of irregular thickness: large cytoplasmic surface, bulging into the sinusoidal lumen, alternating with thin, fenestrated processes *
 - signs of intense activity : numerous, coated and uncoated vesicles, prominent Golgi apparatus, many polysomes and RER profiles, filaments and microtubules *
 - projection of extensions into the lumen, sometimes forming thin fenestrated loops or a complicated network of channels and pouches [5,*]
 - sprouting into the enlarged interhepatocellular space, with occasional formation of complete or incomplete neolumens *

Dividing cells
 - many small mitochondria, several small cytoplasmic vacuoles surrounded by a cytoplasm rich in ribosomes

MORPHOLOGY OF PERISINUSOIDAL CELLS [6,*]
Proliferation of PSC : basal ≈ 3.8% ; 2 days after PH : 26% ; 4 days after PH : 4%
 - the number of lipocytes (expressed per 100 liver cells) increased slightly 2 days after PH
 - vit A (nmol/liver) increased slightly 1 day after PH
 - proliferation of PSC is independant of hepatic vitamin A level (hypo to hypervitaminosis A)

Morphology (ultrastructure) *
 - a few lipid droplets
 - fibroblastic aspect with numerous dilated RER profiles
 - some thickened, discontinuous processes, near to endothelial sprouts

[1] Shinya et al. ,1990 ; [2] Fly & Yu, 1990 [3] Widmann & Fahimi, 1975 ; [4] Widmann & Fahimi, 1976 ; [5] Gendrault et al. ,1986 ; [6] Tanaka et al. ,1991 ; * personnal (unpublished) data

Table 5. LIVER REGENERATION - PARTIAL HEPATECTOMY- ECM (DISSE SPACE) RAT / HUMAN

ADULT LIVER [1]	Collagens	I	III	IV	V	FN	LAM	ENT	Perlecan
DS		+	+	+	+	+	+	+	+
CELLS INVOLVED									
H						++			
PSC		+	+	++	+	+	++	++	
EC		+		+		+	++	+	++
FOETAL LIVER [1,2] H						+	+	+	+
PH [3] PSC						+++			

[1] Clement *et al.*, 1988 [2] Reif *et al.*, 1990 [3] Martinez-Hernandez *et al.*, 1991

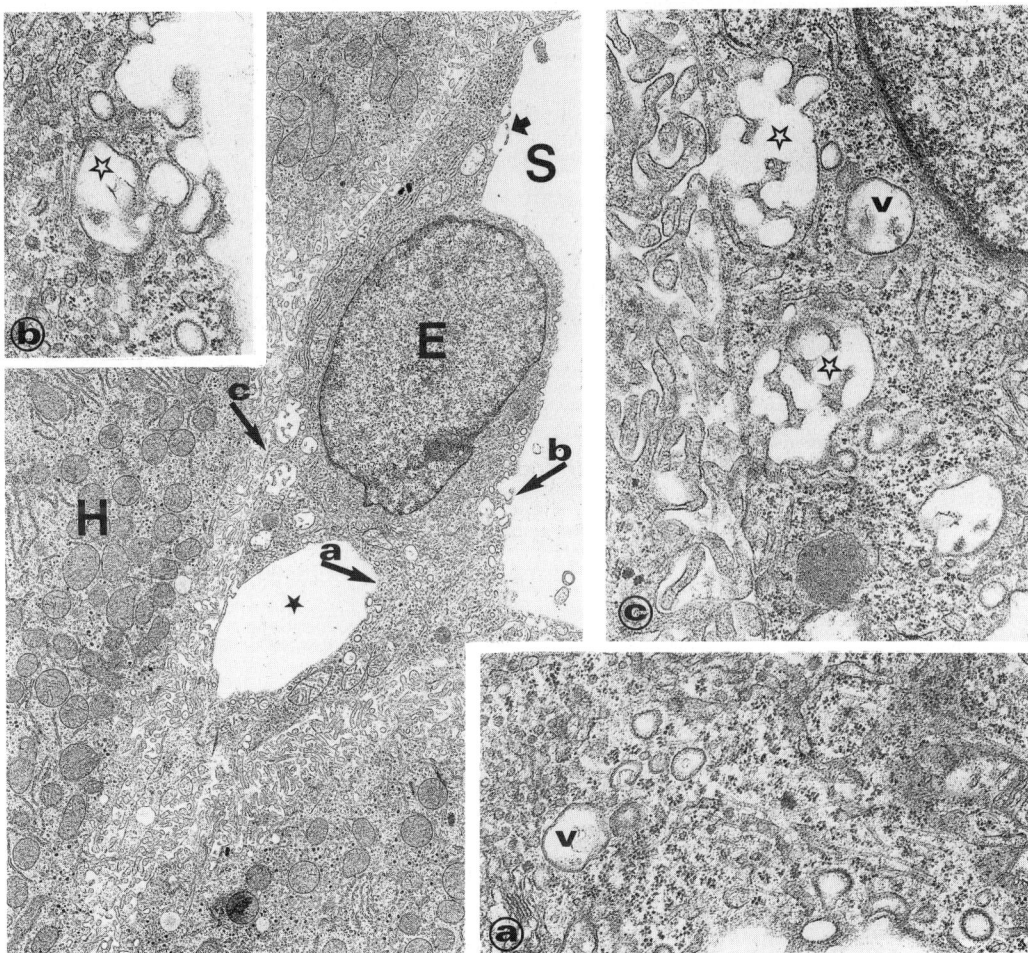

Fig. 2. Two days after 70% hepatectomy in rats - Transmission electron microscopy.
This regenerative endothelial cell (E) shows signs of intense activity, particularly numerous vesicles and vacuoles (V) (inset a). At low and high magnifications (inset b-c), E luminal and abluminal extensions forming fenestrated loops (short arrow), channels and pouches (white star) or luminal cavities (black star) can be seen. These aspects evoke angiogenesis, with extension of E plasma membranes and/or formation of cavities or neolumens from coalescent vesicles and vacuoles.
H: hepatocyte; S: sinusoidal lumen. X 6 500 ; enlargement of different areas of the E : a- c X 27 600

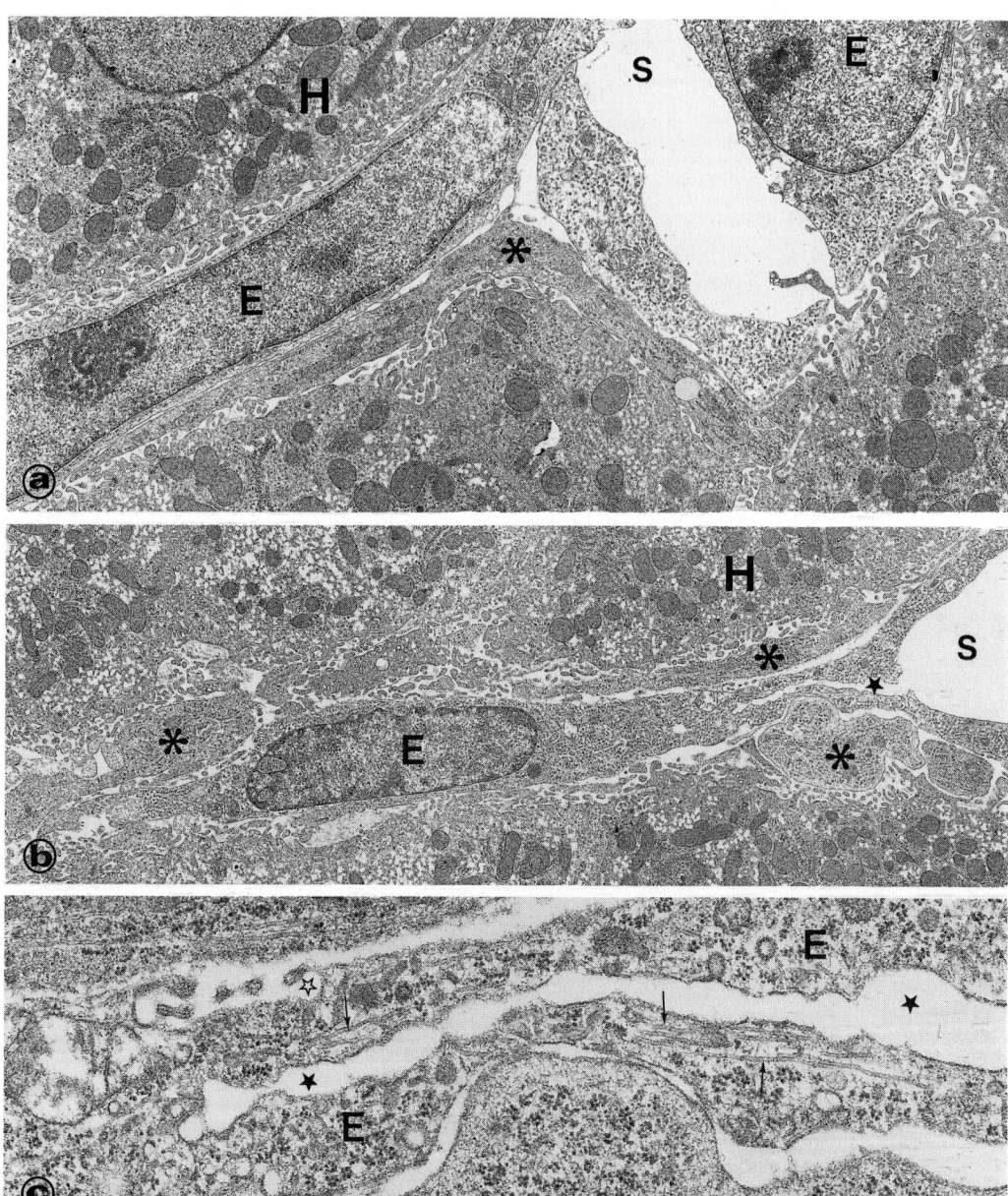

Fig. 3. Two days after 70% hepatectomy in rat - Transmission electron microscopy.
a, b : these endothelial cells (E) which show the cytoplasmic characteristics of intense activity burrow into the enlarged interhepatocellular space.Thick, fibroblastic perisinusoidal cell processes (asterisk) underlie E. c : At a higher magnification of b, the sinusoidal lumen (S) is prolonged by a small canal (black star) which burrows deeper into the cytoplasm of the E. In this area there are numerous microtubules (arrow) and vesicles. The shape of the canal and the proximity of vesicles suggest that it is formed by the coalescence of vesicles with the plasma membrane. On the E abluminal membrane, coalescence of vesicles forms a neolumen (white star).
H: hepatocyte. **a** X 7 400 ; **b** X 5 700; **c** X 31 000

The factors involved in non-parenchymal cell growth have not yet been identified. However it is known that TGF β plays a part in angiogenesis and in the chemotaxis of inflammatory cells and fibroblast proliferation, all of which are processes involved in tissue repair and in control of the synthesis and degradation of the ECM. HGF and EGF are also known to play a role in the growth and chemotaxis of human microvascular endothelial cells in culture (Morimoto *et al.*, 1991). Although the mechanism remains unclear, it has been shown (Rhodin & Fujita, 1989) in the rat mesentery that capillary growth that occurs at the arteriolar-vascular loop follows a well-defined morphological process, in which small endothelial extensions penetrate the basal lamina, evolve into cellular protrusions and develop further into endothelial spurs and short sprouts. These sprouts gradually lengthen : one endothelial cell moves forward followed by a second, elongated bipolar EC, in a sliding, overlapping motion. A small slit-like lumen then emerges and enlarges between the EC. It has also been shown that these long endothelial extensions contain a highly vesicular Golgi area and numerous vesicles, filaments and microtubules.

III-MORPHOLOGY OF NON-PARENCHYMAL CELLS AND OF THE ECM IN HUMANS

We know that the liver regenerates after PH and after orthotopic liver transplantation when the graft implanted is too small. There is, however, no ultrastructural data available on the regenerative process. We have studied regeneration in other models (Table 2). Since results obtained are similar to those obtained in rats after PH, we have outlined only some specific points (Table 6) (Fig. 4, 5).

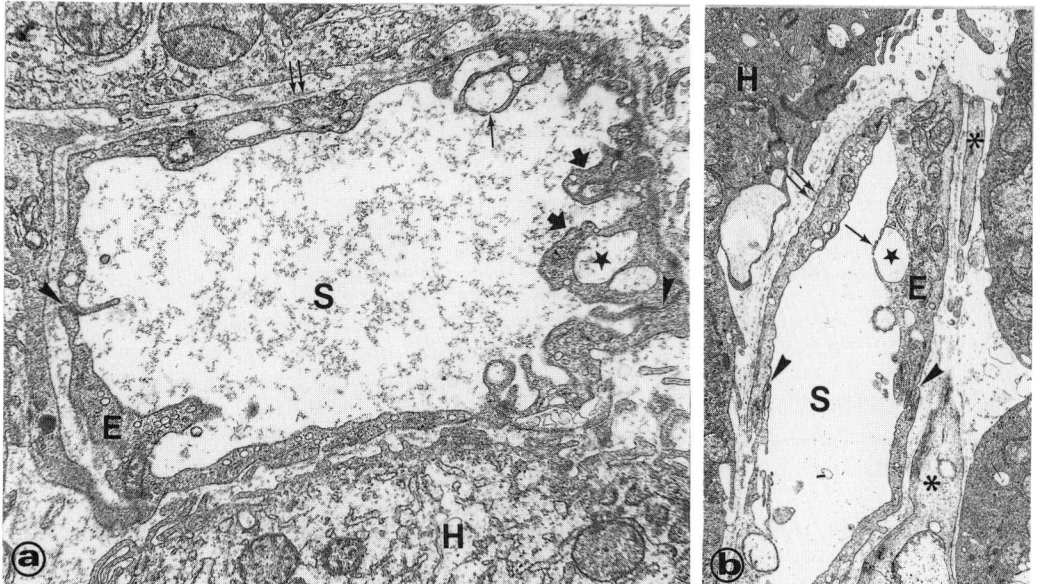

Fig. 4. Human liver - Transmission electron microscopy.
a : hepatocellular adenoma - b : hepatocellular carcinoma.
These endothelial cells (E) project numerous extensions, some fenestrated (thin arrow), some not (thick arrow), into the sinusoidal lumen (S) forming cavities (star). E processes overlap and are occasionally joined by junctional complexes (arrow head). In the enlarged Disse space, basement membranes (double arrow) and thick perisinusoidal processes (asterisk) can be seen.
H: hepatocyte. **a** X 12 500; **b** X 8 500

**Table 6. MORPHOLOGICAL MODIFICATIONS OF SINUSOIDAL CELLS IN HEPATIC REGENERATION
- Additional aspects in other human models of hepatic regeneration -**

- **IN POSTNECROTIC REGENERATION, NRH AND HEPATOCELLULAR TUMORS (FNH, adenoma, HCC)**
  EC: overlapping of processes, joined by junctional complexes, numerous dense bodies
  KC: form part of the sinusoidal barrier, with deep interdigitations between E and KC (but no real junctional complexes)
  LGL: variable number, often in contact with KC, signs of activity (granules)
  PSC: myofibroblastic aspect
  ECM: increased deposits, basement membrane (fragments or continuous)
- **IN REGENERATIVE CIRRHOTIC NODULES**
  sinusoids, compressed between hepatocytes, were occasionally normal or showed varying degrees of abnormality- *regenerative aspects* : cellular fragments some well- defined, others less, form "neo-sinusoids" in between the sinusoidal poles of hepatocytes.

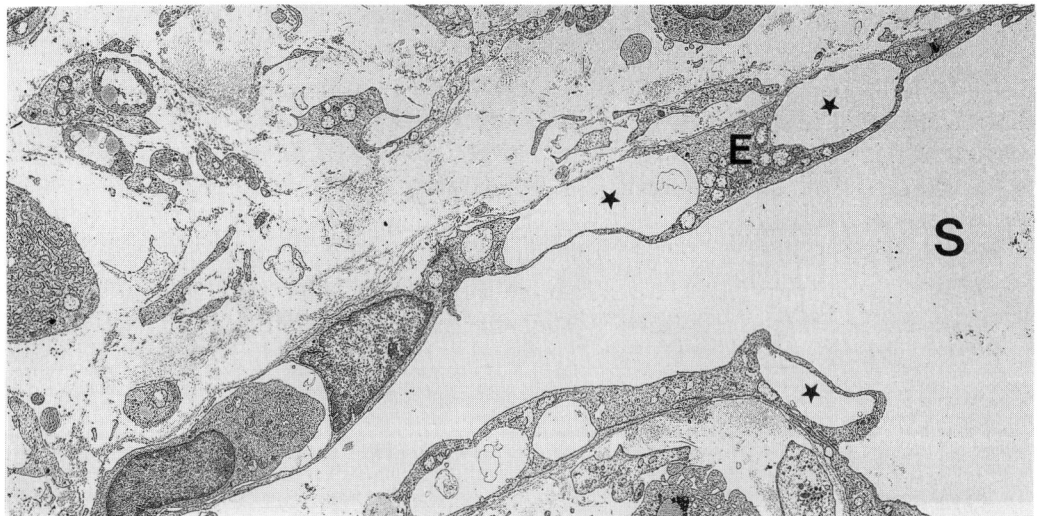

Fig. 5. Human liver - Fulminant hepatitis (amanita phaloides) - Transmission electron microscopy.
In this necrotic centrolobular area, the endothelial barrier (E) around the sinusoidal lumen (S) is preserved. In E cell body and processes, there are several neolumens (black star) of varying size which can be open or closed. X 3 100.

CONCLUSION

The process of liver regeneration involves the regrowth of hepatocytes and sinusoidal cells, the latter with a delay of approximately 24 hours. Much less is known of the mechanisms controlling sinusoidal cell growth. However it is likely that, as for hepatocytes (Fausto, 1990), there are paracrine and autocrine loops controlling this growth (Chen *et al.*, 1990; Meyer *et al.*, 1990). The interaction between hepatocytes and sinusoidal cells is perhaps best illustrated by the concept of the liver as a bioecological system. Liver function is the result of this complex interaction, each cell (hepatocytes, individual non-parenchymal cells and biliary cells) interacting with all the others and with the ECM (Rojkind & Greenwell, 1990). A clear demonstration of this interaction was provided by Kusano (1982) with the injection of isolated hepatocytes into the rat spleen, which then proliferated and reconstituted a hepatic sinusoidal structure.

AKNOWLEDGEMENTS

This work was made possible through grants from the Conseil Régional d'Aquitaine, le Comité de la Dordogne de la ligue contre le Cancer et la Fondation de France pour la Recherche. The authors wish to thank L. Boussarie, P. Gonzalez and Maïté Munoz for their excellent technical assistance.

REFERENCES

Andus, T., Bauer, J., and Gerok, W. (1991) : Effects of cytokines on the liver. In *Hepatology* 13, 364-375

Bioulac-Sage, P., Lamouliatte, H., Saric, J., Merlio, J.P., and Balabaud, C. (1986) : Ultrastructure of sinusoidal cells in a benign liver cell adenoma. *Ultrastruct. Pathol.* 10, 49-54.

Bioulac-Sage, P., Lafon, M.E., Le Bail, B., Boulard, A., Dubuisson, L., Quinton A., Lamouliatte, H., Saric, J., Balabaud, C. (1988) : Ultrastructure of sinusoids in liver disease. In *Sinusoids in human liver: health and disease*, eds P. Bioulac-Sage, C. Balabaud, pp. 223-278. Rijswijk : Kupffer Cell Foundation.

Bioulac-Sage, P., Dubuisson, L., Bedin, C., Gonzalez, P., and Balabaud, C.(1992a): Selenium induced liver damage : cirrhosis or nodular regenerative hyperplasia ? In *Cellular and Molecular Aspects of Cirrhosis*, eds B. Clement and A. Guillouzo, Vol 216, pp 77-80. Montrouge : John Libbey Eurotext

Bioulac-Sage, P., Le Bail, B., Carles, J., Bernard, P., Janvier, G., Brechenmacher, C., Saric, J., Balabaud, C., and the PATH group (1992b): Ultrastructure of sinusoids in human cirrhotic nodules. In *Cellular and Molecular Aspects of Cirrhosis*, eds B. Clement and A. Guillouzo, Vol 216, pp 91-101. Montrouge : John Libbey Eurotext.

Blouin, A., Bolender, R.P., Weibel, E.W. (1977) : Distribution of organelles and membranes between hepatocytes and non-hepatocytes in the rat liver parenchyma. A stereological study. *J. Cell. Biol.* 72, 441-455

Callea, F., Brissigotti, M., Fabbretti G., Sciot, R., Van Eyken, P., Favret M. (1991) : Cirrhosis of the-liver. A regenerative process. *Dig. Dis. Sc.* 36, 1287-1293

Chen, W., Steffan, A.M., Braunwald, J., Nonnenmacher, H., Kirn, A., Gendrault, J.L. (1990) : Inhibition in fat-storing cell multiplication by a factor produced by normal cultured murine hepatocytes. *J. Hepatol.* 11, 330-338

Clément, B., Rescan, PY., Baffet, G., Loréal, O., Lehry, D., Campion, JP., Guillouzo, A. (1988) : Hepatocytes may produce laminin in fibrotic liver and in primary culture. *Hepatology* 8 : 794-803

Fausto, N. (1990) : Hepatic Regeneration. In *Hepatology. A text book of liver disease*, eds. Zakim D, Boyer T.D., pp. 49-65. Philadelphia : W.B. Saunders Company.

Flye, M.W., and Yu, S. (1990) : Augmentation of cell-mediated cytotoxicity following 50% partial hepatectomy. *Transplantation* 49, 81-587

Francavilla, A., Starzl, T.E, Porter, K., Scotti Foglieni, C., Michalopoulos, G.K., Carrieri, G., Trejo J., Azzarone, A., Barone, M., Hua Zeng, Q. (1991) : Screening for candidate hepatic growth factors by selective portal infusion after canine Eck's fistula. *Hepatology* 14 , 665-670

Gendrault, J.L., Gut, J.P. (1986) : Glucan-treatment of frog virus 3 infected mice. A model for liver sinusoid regeneration. In *Cells of the Hepatic Sinusoid,* eds. Kirn A., Knook D.L., Wisse E., pp. 357-362. Rijswijk : Kupffer Cell Foundation.

Kawakita, N., Seki, S., Sakaguchi, H., Yanai, A., Kuroki, T., Mizoguchi, Y., Kobayashi, K., Monna, T. Kaneda, K. (1991) : Analysis of the proliferative sinusoidal cells in patients with confluent hepatic necrosis. In *Cells and the Hepatic Sinusoid*, Vol. 3, ed. E. Wisse, D.L. Knook, R.S. McCuskey, pp. 242-244. The Nehterlands: Kupffer Cell Foundation.

Kusano, M., Mito, M. (1982) : Observations on the fine structure of long-survived isolated hepatocytes inoculated into rat spleen. *Gastroenterology* 82 , 616-628

Martinez-Hernandez, A., Martinez-Delgado, F. (1991) : The extracellular matrix in hepatic regeneration. Localization of collagen types I, III, IV, laminin, and fibronectin. *Lab. Invest.* 64 , 157-166

Meyer, D.H., Bachem, M.G., Gressner, A.M. (1990) : Transformed fat storing cells inhibit the proliferation of cultured hepatocytes by secretion of transforming growth factor beta. *J. Hepatol.* 11, 86-91

Michalopoulos, G.K.& Zarnegar R(1992) : Liver regeneration : molecular mechanisms of growth control. *FASEB* 4 , 176-186

Morimoto, A., Okamura, K. , Hamanaka, R., Sato, Y.(1991) : Hepatocyte growth factor modulates migration and proliferation of human microvascular endothelial cells in culture. *Biochem. Biophys. Res. Com.* 179 , 1042-1049

Nakatsukasa, H., Evarts, R.P., Hsia, CC., Thorgeirsson S.S. (1990) : Transforming growth factor-β1 and type I procollagen transcripts during regeneration and early fibrosis of rat liver. *Lab. Invest.* 63 , 171-180

Noji, S., Tashiro, K. Koyama, E., Nohno, T., Ohyama K., Taniguchi, S., Nakamura, T. (1990) :Expression of hepatocyte growth factor gene in endothelial and Kupffer cells of damaged rat livers, as revealed by in situ hybridization. *Biochem. Biophys. Res. Com.* 173 , 42-43.

Reif, S., Terranova, V.P., El-Bendary, M., Lebenthal, E., Petell, J.K. (1990) : Modulation of extracellular matrix proteins in rat liver during development. *Hepatology* 12 , 519-525

Rhodin, J.A.G., Fujita, H. (1989) : Capillary growth in the mesentery of normal young rats. Intravital video and electron microscope analyses. *J. Submicrosc. Cytol. Pathol.* 21 , 1-34

Rojkind, M., and Greenwel, P. (1988). The liver as a bioecological system. In *The Liver : Biology and Pathology*, ed. I.M. Arias, W.B. Jakoby, H. Popper, D. Schachter, and D.A. Shafritz, pp 1269-1285. New York : Raven Press Ltd.

Seki, S., Sakaguchi, H., Kawakita, N., Yanai, A., Kuroki, T., Mizoguchi, Y., Kobayashi, K., Monna, T. (1991) : Detection of proliferating liver cells in various diseases by a monoclonal antibody against DNA polymerase-α : with special reference to the relationship between hepatocytes and sinusoidal cells. *Hepatology* 14 , 781-788

Shinya, M., Kaneda, K., Wake, K., Yokomuro, K. (1990) : Large granular lymphocytes and Kupffer cells in regenerating rat liver. *Biomed. Res.* 11, 199-206

Schirmacher, P., Geerts, A., Pietrangelo, A., Dienes, H.P., Rogler, C.E. (1992) : Hepatocyte growth factor/hepatopoietin A is expressed in fat-storing cells from rat liver but not myofibroblast-like cells derived from fat-storing cells. *Hepatology* 15 , 5-11

Tabarin, A., Bioulac-Sage, P., Merlio, J.P., Lamouliatte, H., Saric, J., and Balabaud, C. (1986) Sinusoids ultrastructure of human hepatocellular carcinoma. *J. Submicros. Cytol.* 18 , 171-176

Tanaka, Y., Mak, K.M., Lieber, C.S. (1990) : Immunohistochemical detection of proliferating lipocytes in regenerating rat liver. *J. Pathol.* 160 , 129-134

Widmann, J.J., Fahimi, H.D. (1975) : Proliferation of mononuclear phagocytes (Kupffer cells) and endothelial cells in regenerating rat liver. A light and electron microscopic cytochemical study. *Am. J. Pathol.* 80, 349-360

Widmann, J.J. and Fahimi, H. (1976) : Proliferation of endothelial cells in estrogen-stimulated rat liver. A light and Electron microscopic cytochemical study. *Lab. Invest.* 34 , 141-149.

Wolf, H.K., Zarnegar, R., Michalopoulos, G.K. (1991) : Localization of hepatocyte growth factor in human and rat tissues : an immunohistochemical study. *Hepatology* 14 , 488-494

Zindy, F., Lamas, E., Schmidt, S., Kim, A., Brechot, C. (1992) : Expression of insulin-like growth factor II (IGF-II) and IGF-II, IGF-I and insulin receptors mRNAs in isolated non-parenchymal rat liver cells. *J. Hepatol.* 14 , 30-34

Ito cell proliferation *in vivo* and *in vitro*

Jean Rosenbaum, Frédéric Charlotte*

INSERM U.99 and *Departement d'Anatomie et Cytologie Pathologiques, Hôpital Henri Mondor, 94010 Créteil, France

Ito cells (also called lipocytes, stellate cells, perisinusoidal cells or fat-storing cells) are located in the space of Disse between endothelial cells and hepatocytes. They have been initially recognized as the main storage site for vitamin A. However, in the past 10 years, their role in the pathophysiology of hepatic fibrosis has been firmly established. More recently, several other functions of Ito cells, including a potential role in hepatic regeneration and contractile properties suggesting a role in liver vasoregulation have been demonstrated. This paper will focus on Ito cells in liver fibrosis and regeneration.

ITO CELL PROLIFERATION IN FIBROSIS

A- Experimental models

Ito cell proliferation can be triggered experimentally by several agents that induce diffuse liver fibrosis such as carbon tetrachloride (CCl_4), dimethylnitrosamine and ethanol but also in localized hepatic injury as will be discussed below.

1- CCl_4 intoxication

Acute administration of CCl_4 to rats or mice leads to a rapid necrosis of centrilobular hepatocytes associated with a marked mononuclear infiltrate in the same area. These changes begin to resolve from day 4 onwards. If CCl_4 is administered chronically, fibrosis develops starting from centrilobular areas and culminating in cirrhosis after 4 to 6 weeks of treatment.

After a single CCl_4 injection, the number of Ito cells increases several fold in the centrilobular area with a peak at 72-96 h post-injection (Burt *et al.*, 1986; Geerts *et al.*, 1991). No increase is apparent in periportal areas. The mechanisms responsible for the increased Ito cell number are likely to involve recruitment of Ito cells in the centrilobular areas rather than cell multiplication. This is evidenced by the lack of significant [^{3}H] thymidine incorporation into Ito cells during the first 48 hours (Geerts *et al.*, 1991). The recruitment of Ito cells is probably due to the release of chemotactic mediators by inflammatory cells infiltrating the area. Several possible candidates have been identified including platelet-derived growth factor (PDGF) (Pinzani *et al.*, 1990b), transforming growth factor ß1 (TGFß1) (Nakatsukasa *et al.*, 1990), tumor necrosis factor alpha (Armendariz Borunda *et al.*, 1991) and basic fibroblast growth factor (bFGF) (Charlotte *et al.*, 1991).

In the course of chronic CCl_4 intoxication, Ito cells increase in number in areas linking centrilobular veins where fibrosis will ultimately develop. This increase is due to cell multiplication as evidenced by the presence of mitotic figures, a high thymidine index (Geerts *et al.*, 1991), or intake of bromodeoxyuridine (Tanaka *et al.*, 1991). A very important feature is that these changes are paralleled by dramatic phenotypic modifications of Ito cells. These include a diminution in vitamin A content, a large increase in the rough endoplasmic reticulum area, apparition of a large number of microfilaments bundles together with neoexpression of alpha-smooth muscle-specific actin. This new phenotype is regarded as transitional, activated, or myofibroblast-like and is associated with an increased production of fibrosis components by the cells (McGee & Patrick, 1972; Tanaka *et al.*, 1991).

2- Dimethylnitrosamine intoxication.
Like CCl_4 intoxication, dimethylnitrosamine intoxication leads to cirrhosis within a few weeks (Jezequel *et al.*, 1990). As described in the CCl_4 model, the number of Ito cells exhibiting a transitional phenotype also increases in the fibrous septae.

3- Ethanol.
Rats fed ethanol together with a high fat-low protein diet develop fibrosis in a high proportion of cases (French *et al.*, 1988). In this model, there is an increase in Ito cell number in the fibrous septae. These Ito cells exhibit the activated phenotype. Interestingly, even lobular Ito cells that do not participate in fibrous septa formation show this activated phenotype, thus suggesting that factors other than those inducing phenotypic changes are necessary for the increased fibrogenic activity.

4- Focal hepatic lesion.
Creation of a focal liver lesion with a liquid nitrogen-cooled needle leads to a sequence of events that mimicks to an extent those induced by acute CCl_4 intoxication. Twenty four hours following the lesion, the damaged site is infiltrated by inflammatory cells, followed on the next days by an influx of Ito cells that are probably again attracted by chemotactic factors originating from the inflammatory cells (Ogawa *et al.*, 1986).

B- Human studies

These studies have met with the difficulty of an easy identification of human Ito cells in tissue sections. Whereas desmin is a reliable marker of Ito cells in the rat, its use a a marker of human Ito cells is controversial. We have however unpublished evidence that lobular Ito cells from normal human liver stain for desmin. We have also observed, as others (Schmitt-Gräff *et al.*, 1991) that many desmin-positive cells were demonstrable in fibrous septae during chronic liver disease. Electron microscopic studies have shown that in the course of chronic alcoholic disease, the number of typical Ito cells decreases, while the number of transitional cells increases (Mak & Lieber, 1988; Horn *et al.*, 1986; Minato *et al.*, 1983). This is associated with the appearance of alpha-smooth muscle-specific actin staining in the centrilobular and fibrotic areas (Schmitt-Gräff *et al.*, 1991; Nouchi *et al.*, 1991). Taken together, these data suggest that in man as in rat, at least a part of the transitional cells from fibrous

septae derive from Ito cells through transformation and proliferation.
Apart from alcoholic liver disease, increased Ito cell numbers are also found in a number of diffuse or focal human liver diseases (Schmitt-Gräff *et al.*, 1991).

C- *In vitro* studies

As for the *in vivo* studies, most data come from animal (mainly rat) experiments. Many soluble factors have been shown to influence Ito cell proliferation, together with extracellular matrix components. We will specially focus on the role of autocrine and paracrine mediators as they appear to play a major role.

1- Kupffer cell-derived factors.
Several groups have shown that Kupffer cell (KC) conditioned medium had profound effects on rat Ito cells : a) it stimulates transformation of fat-laden Ito cells to myofibroblasts (MF) ; b) it stimulates proliferation, collagen and proteoglycan synthesis of Ito cells (Armendariz-Borunda *et al.*, 1989; Bachem *et al.*, 1992a ; Friedman & Arthur, 1989 ; Meyer *et al.*, 1990 ; Shiratori *et al.*, 1986). These activities are mediated by several soluble factors produced by KC. Evidence implicates **TGFß1** as one of the major mediator from KC: 1) TGFß1 mimicks the effect of conditioned medium in stimulating the transdifferentiation of Ito cells into MF and increasing their collagen and proteoglycan synthesis; 2) KC express TGFß1 mRNA and protein ; 3) The effect of KC conditioned medium on these parameters is abrogated in the presence of anti-TGFß antibody. It is interesting to note that TGFß1 mRNA was increased in KC isolated from alcohol-fed (Matsuoka & Tsukamoto, 1990) or D-galactosamine treated rats (Meyer *et al.*, 1990) *vs* normal rats, both conditions being associated with activation of Ito cells. On the other hand, TGFß1 has a growth inhibitory effect on rat Ito cells (Davis, 1988) which means that KC conditioned medium must also contain growth promoting agents. Part of the mitogenic activity is likeky due to secretion of **TGF-alpha** since KC express TGF-alpha mRNA and protein (Meyer *et al.*,1990) and that TGF-alpha is mitogenic for Ito cells (Bachem *et al.*, 1989). Additionnally, KC secrete an as yet uncharacterized low molecular weight factor that **induces PDGFß receptor expression** on rat Ito cells, making them susceptible to the effect of PDGF (Friedman & Arthur,1989). PDGF is apparently not secreted by KC themselves but it could be released from platelets during degranulation at the site of liver injury, or, as shown in the guinea pig, from sinusoidal endothelial cells (Rieder *et al.*, 1992). Finally, KC from CCl$_4$-treated rats secrete **tumor necrosis factor alpha** (Armendariz-Borunda *et al.*,1991) that has been shown to enhance the transdifferentiating effect of TGFß1 on Ito cells (Bachem *et al.*,1992b).

These accumulated evidences point out to a major pathophysiological role for KC or macrophage-derived products in Ito cell activation and proliferation. This is even more likely given the close anatomical association between these cell types in the course of fibrogenesis.

2- Liver myofibroblast-derived factors.
Ito cells in their MF phenotype synthetize several growth factors that can stimulate quiescent Ito cells to transdifferentiate in MF and proliferate. Bachem *et al.* (1992a) have shown that MF synthetized both **TGFß1** (that induces transdifferentiation) and **TGF-alpha** (that is mitogenic for Ito cells). However, the mitogenic activity of MF conditioned medium was only partially suppressed by anti-TGF-alpha antibody, suggesting that MF synthetized other growth factors. This is supported by results of Pinzani *et al.* (1990a) demonstrating that MF synthetize and respond to **insulin-like growth factor I**.

Furthermore, we have shown that rat MF also synthetized **bFGF** that stimulates their own growth (Rosenbaum *et al.*,1991, unpublished results). Synthesis of such an array of growth regulators could be a key factor in the self perpetuation of Ito cell activation and proliferation in liver diseases.

3- Role of endothelial cell- and hepatocyte-derived factors.
The role of **endothelial cells** in the control of Ito cell proliferation could be complex as these cells have been shown to synthetize several growth regulators with apparent opposite effects. We have shown that mouse liver endothelial cells synthetize a bFGF-related molecule (Rosenbaum *et al.*, 1989a) that is mitogenic for Ito cells, while they also secrete a growth inhibitor for these cells (Rosenbaum *et al.*, 1989b). Further, as discussed above, guinea pig liver endothelial cells secrete a PDGF isoform that is mitogenic for Ito cells (Rieder *et al.*, 1992). The actual role of sinusoidal endothelial cells will be more clearly defined when more is known about *in vivo* expression of these molecules in various pathophysiological settings.

Mouse **hepatocytes** secrete constitutively an inhibitor for Ito cells (Chen *et al.*, 1990). It is suggested that diseased hepatocytes (in this case, hepatocytes infected with ectromelia virus) are no more able to produce this compound. This could lead to Ito cell proliferation in the *in vivo* situation. On the other hand, hepatocytes may also promote Ito cell proliferation in some circumstances through secretion of TGF-alpha (Mead & Fausto, 1989).

4- Extracellular matrix.
The substrate on which Ito cells are grown plays an important role in controlling the growth and differentiation of these cells. Friedman *et al.* (1989) showed that if freshly isolated rat Ito cells were cultured on a complex basement matrix, they retained their initial characteristics, while culture on plain plastic leaded to transdifferentiation in MF. In the same line, Davis (1988) showed that when Ito cells were grown on type IV collagen (supposed to be part of their normal environment in the intact healthy liver), they did not increase their collagen synthesis in response to TGFß1, while cells grown on type I collagen (a composant of the abnormal liver matrix during fibrogenesis) responded to TGFß1. In this context, the secretion of a type IV collagenase by KC and Ito cells might be relevant as breakdown of the normal type IV matrix could facilitate Ito cell activation by soluble mediators (Arthur *et al.*, 1989).

5- Particularities of human Ito cells
Human Ito cells can be isolated in their vitamin A-rich phenotype from perfusion of large pieces of human liver (Friedman *et al.*, 1990). They can also be isolated in MF phenotype by culture of liver explants (Rosenbaum *et al.*, 1991). While the response of human liver MF to several growth factors (bFGF, PDGF-AB, epidermal growth factor/TGF-alpha) is similar to what is observed with rat cells (Rosenbaum *et al.*, 1991), several distinctive features are obvious. TGFß1 which is is antiproliferative for rat Ito cells is a potent mitogenic factor for human MF (Win *et al.*, 1991). Evidence suggests that this mitogenic effect is at least in part due to autocrine production of PDGF-A chain by TGFß1-stimulated MF themselves. This points out to 2 other differences between rat and human cells : human cells secrete PDGF while rat ones do not (Pinzani *et al.*, 1991); human cells respond to PDGF-AA although rat cells do not as they lack the alpha-type PDGF receptor (Heldin *et al.*, 1991). These differences must lead to caution when extrapolating results obtained with rat Ito cells to human ones.

6- Temptative integration of events occuring in rat liver fibrogenesis.

The mechanisms described in the previous paragraphs are depicted schematically in Fig.1.

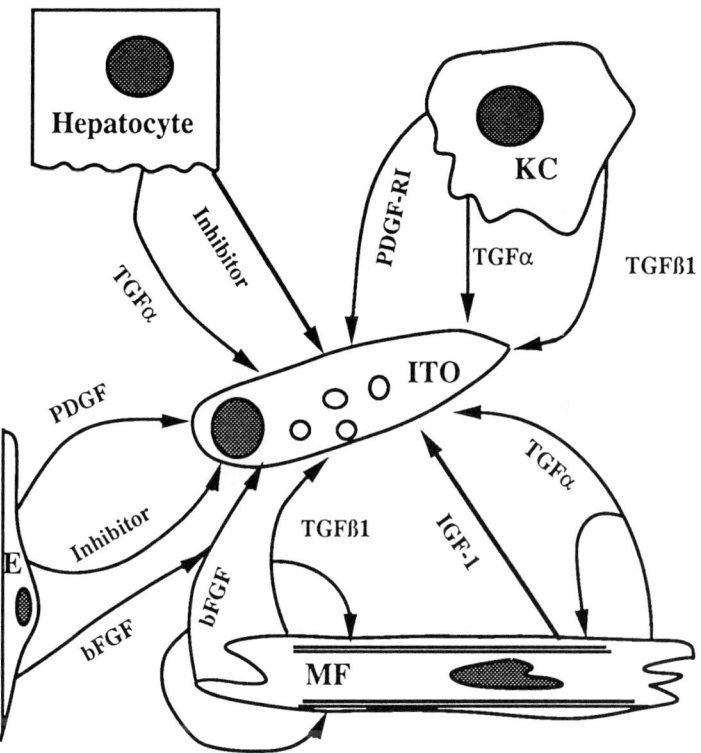

Fig.1 Postulated mechanisms of activation of Ito cells in liver fibrosis. At the initial stage of liver injury, KC or activated macrophages can induce transdifferentiation of Ito cells *via* TGFß1 and proliferation through secretion of TGF alpha and the PDGF receptor inducer (PDGF-RI). Then, sustained activation could be due to MF-derived factors. Hepatocytes and endothelial cells (E) could modulate this process.

7- Modulation of Ito cell transdifferentiation and proliferation.

As one of the most obvious feature of transdifferentiation of Ito cells is the loss of intracellular vitamin A, it was logical to test the effects of vitamin A and its derivatives on Ito cell functions. Davis & Vucic (1988) showed that exposure of liver MF to exogenous retinol inhibited Ito cell proliferation. Retinoic acid was even more potent and also decreased collagen production (Davis *et al.*, 1990). However, none of these mediators did induce a reversion to the original phenotype nor reduce alpha smooth muscle-specific actin expression.

Gamma-interferon added to freshly isolated Ito cells prevented largely the appearance of 2 markers of transdifferentiation, *i.e.*, smooth muscle actin and collagen type I expression (Rockey *et al.*, 1991). It might prove valuable to test associations of retinoids with γ-interferon.

It is worth noting that both these compounds have demonstrated antifibrogenic activity *in vivo* in experimental models of liver fibrosis (Senoo & Wake, 1985; Czaja *et al.*, 1989).

ITO CELLS AND LIVER REGENERATION

Two aspects must be considered :
- the proliferation of Ito cells during liver regeneration;
- their participation in the regenerative process.

A- Proliferation of Ito cells during liver regeneration

Like every cell type in the liver, Ito cells proliferate in response to 2/3 hepatectomy in the rat. The kinetics of this process have been studied by means of double staining with anti-desmin and anti-bromodeoxyuridine antibody (Tanaka *et al.*, 1990). This study showed a peak proliferation at 48-72 hours, well after hepatocyte peak DNA synthesis. This lag between hepatocytes and non parenchymal cell regeneration had already been noted (Widmann & Fashimi, 1975; Martinez-Hernandez *et al.*, 1991). It suggests that hepatocytes and non parenchymal cells (among them Ito cells) do not proliferate in response to the same stimuli. The stimulus for Ito cell proliferation could actually come from regenerating hepatocytes that have been shown to express several growth factors, notably TGF alpha (Mead & Fausto, 1989) and acidic FGF (Kan *et al.*, 1989).

An important characteristic of Ito cell proliferation during liver regeneration is that it occurs without accumulation of Ito cells at a single site and without concomitant fibrosis deposition, showing again that proliferative and fibrogenic activities can be dissociated in Ito cells.

B- Role of Ito cells in the regenerative process

This area is still an open field. There are however two types of data suggesting that Ito cells play an active part in the regenerative process.

Martinez-Hernandez *et al.* (1991) showed that Ito cells were responsible for the increased sinusoidal laminin staining observed transiently in the few days following 2/3 hepatectomy. In regard to the well-known role of laminin in the attachment and differentiation of hepatocytes, it is likely that Ito cells, through laminin expression, help promoting liver regeneration.

Very recently, Ito cells were shown to be a major source of hepatocyte growth factor (HGF) in rat liver (Maher, 1991; Schirmacher *et al.*, 1991). HGF is thought to be the first agent that initiates hepatocyte proliferation during regeneration and it has also been identified as a major growth factor for biliary epithelial cells (Joplin *et al.*, 1992). Ito cell secretion of HGF could thus be a key factor in the initiation of liver regeneration. Very interestingly, it was shown that whether freshly isolated Ito cells expressed HGF, cells that had differentiated into MF did no more express it (Schirmacher *et al.*, 1991). This would suggest a limited supply of HGF in the fibrotic liver where MF predominate over typical Ito cells.

CONCLUSION

Ito cell proliferation accompanies both fibrogenesis and liver regeneration. The main difference between the 2 situations is that while during fibrogenesis Ito cells accumulate at specific sites and deposit fibrosis components, during regeneration, Ito cells proliferate harmoniously without permanently depositing fibrosis components. The molecular basis of Ito cell proliferation are beginning to be understood : paracrine/autocrine activation seems to be particularly important. Studies dealing with the modulation of transdifferentiation and proliferation of Ito cells yield encouraging results notably with retinoids and γ-interferon and this should certainly be an area of future intense research together with studies aiming at reducing the fibrogenic potential of Ito cells.

REFERENCES

Armendariz-Borunda, J., Greenwell, P.,& Rojkind, M. (1989): Kupffer cells from CCl_4-treated rat livers induce skin fibroblast and liver fat-storing cell proliferation in culture. *Matrix 9*: 150-158.

Armendariz-Borunda, J., Seyer, J.M., Postlethwaite, A.E.,& Kang, A.H. (1991): Kupffer cells from carbon tetrachloride-injured rat livers produce chemotactic factors for fibroblasts and monocytes. The role of tumor necrosis α. *Hepatology 14*: 895-900.

Arthur, M.J.P., Friedman, S.L., Roll, F.J.,& Bissell D.M.(1989): Lipocytes from normal rat liver release a neutral metalloproteinase that degrades basement membrane (type IV) collagen. *J. Clin. Invest. 84*: 1076-1085.

Bachem, M.G., Riess, U.,& Gressner AM.(1989): Liver fat storing cell proliferation is stimulated by epidermal growth factor/transforming growth factor alpha and inhibited by transforming growth factor ß. *Biochem. Biophys. Res. Commun.162*: 708-714.

Bachem, M.G, Meyer, D., Melchior, R., Sell, K.M., & Gressner, A.M. (1992a): Activation of rat liver perisinusoidal lipocytes by transforming growth factors derived from myofibroblastlike cells. A potential mechanism of self perpetuation in liver fibrogenesis. *J. Clin. Invest. 89*: 19-27.

Bachem, M.G., Melchior, R.J.,& Gressner A.M. (1992b):Activation of perisinusoidal lipocytes (transdifferentiation into myofibroblast-like cells) is stimulated by transforming growth factor ß1 (TGFß1) and tumor necrosis factor alpha (TNFα). In *International Falk Symposium: Molecular and Cell Biology of Liver Fibrogenesis*, Marburg.

Burt, A.D., Robertson, J.L., Heir, J.,& Macsween, N.M. (1986): Desmin-containing stellate cells in rat liver; distribution in normal animals and response to experimental acute liver injury. *J. Pathol. 150*: 29-35.

Charlotte, F., Win, K.M., Mallat, A., Preaux, A.M., Dhumeaux, D., Zafrani, E.S., Mavier, P.,& Rosenbaum, J. (1991): Immunohistochemical study of the expression of basic fibroblast growth factor (bFGF) in normal rat liver and carbon tetrachloride-induced fibrosis [Abstract]. *Hepatology 14*: 183A.

Chen, W., Steffan, A.M., Braunwald, J., Nonenmacher, H., Kirn, A.,& Gendrault, J.L. (1990): Inhibition in fat-storing cell multiplication by a factor produced by normal cultured murine hepatocytes. *J. Hepatol. 11*: 330-338.

Czaja, M.J., Weiner, F.R., Takahashi, S., Giambrone, M.A., Van der Meide, P.H., Schellekens, H., Biempica, L.,& Zern, M.A. (1989): γ-interferon treatment inhibits collagen deposition in murine schistosomiasis. *Hepatology 10*: 795-800.

Davis, B.H. (1988): Transforming growth factor ß responsiveness is modulated by the extracellular collagen matrix during hepatic Ito cell culture. *J. Cell. Physiol. 136*: 547-553.

Davis, B.H.,& Vucic, A. (1988): The effect of retinol on Ito cell proliferation *in vitro*. *Hepatology 8*: 788-793.

Davis, B.H., Kramer, R.T.,& Davidson, N.O. (1990): Retinoic acid modulates rat Ito cell proliferation, collagen, and transforming growth factor ß production. *J. Clin. Invest. 86*: 2062-2070.

French, S.W., Miyamoto, K., Wong, K., Jui, L.,& Briere, L.(1988): Role of the Ito cell in liver parenchymal fibrosis in rats fed alcohol and a high fat-low protein diet. *Am. J. Pathol. 132*: 73-85.

Friedman, S.L., Roll, F.J., Boyles, J., Arenson, D.M.,& Bissell, D.M.(1989): Maintenance of differentiated phenotype of cultured rat hepatic lipocytes by basement membrane matrix. *J. Biol. Chem. 264*: 10756-10762.

Friedman, S.L.,& Arthur, M.J.P. (1989): Activation of cultured rat hepatic lipopcytes by Kupffer cell conditioned medium. Direct enhancement of matrix synthesis and stimulation of cell proliferation via induction of platelet-derived growth factor receptors. *J. Clin. Invest. 84*: 1780-1785.

Friedman, S.L., Rockey, D.C., McGuire, R.F., Boyles, J.K., & Yamasaki, G.(1990): Morphologic and functional studies of human hepatic lipocytes in early primary culture [Abstract]. *Hepatology 12*: 908.

Geerts, A., Lazou, J.M., De Bleser, P.,& Wisse, E.(1991): Tissue distribution, quantitation and proliferation kinetics of fat-storing cells in carbon tetrachloride-injured rat liver. *Hepatology 13*: 1193-1202.

Heldin, P., Pertoft, H., Nordlinder, H., Heldin, CH.,& Laurent, T.C.(1991): Differential expression of platelet-derived growth factor α- and ß- receptors on fat-storing cells and endothelial cells of rat liver. *Exp. Cell. Res. 193*: 364-369.

Horn. T., Junge. J.,& Christoffersen, P.(1986): Early alcoholic liver injury. Activation of lipocytes in acinar zone 3 and correlation to degree of collagen formation in the Disse space. *J. Hepatol. 3* :333-340.

Jezequel, A.M., Ballardini, G., Mancini, R., Paolucci, F., Bianchi, F.B.,& Orlandi, F. (1990): Modulation of extracellular matrix components during dimethylnitrosamine-induced cirrhosis. *J. Hepatol. 11*: 206-214.

Joplin, R., Neuberger, J.M.,& Strain, A.J. (1992): Human biliary epithelial (BEC) cells from normal and primary biliary cirrhotic (PBC) liver proliferate in response to human hepatocyte growth factor (hHGF) in vitro. In *International Falk Symposium: Molecular and Cell Biology of Liver Fibrogenesis*, Marburg.

Kan, M., Huang, J., Mansson, P.E., Yasumitsu, H., Carr, B.,& McKeehan, W.L. (1989): Heparin-binding growth factor type 1(acidic fibroblast growth factor): a potential biphasic autocrine and paracrine regulator of hepatocyte regeneration. *Proc. Natl. Acad. Sci. USA. 86*: 7432-7436.

Maher, J.J. (1991); Hepatocyte growth factor mRNA is localized primarily in lipocytes in normal rat liver and increases in response to carbon tetrachloride [Abstract]. *Hepatology 14*: 95A.

Mak, K.M.,& Lieber, C.S. (1988): Lipocytes and transitional cells in alcoholic liver disease: a morphometric study. *Hepatology 8*: 1027-1033.

Martinez-Hernandez, A., Delgado, F.M.,& Amenta, P.S. (1991): The extracellular matrix in hepatic regeneration. Localization of collagen types I, III, IV, laminin, and fibronectin. *Lab. Invest. 64*: 157-166.

Matsuoka, M.,& Tsukamoto, H. (1990): Stimulation of hepatic lipocyte collagen production by Kupffer cell-derived transforming growth factor ß: implication for a pathogenetic role in alcoholic liver fibrogenesis. *Hepatology 11*: 599-605.

McGee, J.O.D.,& Patrick, R.S.(1972): The role of perisinusoidal cells in hepatic fibrogenesis. An electron microscopic study of acute carbon tetrachloride liver injury. *Lab. Invest. 26*: 429-440.

Mead, J.E.,& Fausto, N. (1989): Transforming growth factor α may be a physiological regulator of liver regeneration by means of an autocrine mechanism. *Proc. Natl. Acad. Sci. USA. 86*: 1558-1562.

Meyer, D.H., Bachem, M.G.,& Gressner, A.M.(1990): Modulation of hepatic lipocyte proteoglycan synthesis and proliferation by Kupffer cell-derived transforming growth factors type ß1 and type α. *Biochem. Biophys. Res. Commun. 171*: 1122-1129.

Minato, Y., Hasumura, Y.,& Takeuchi, J. (1983): The role of fat-storing cells in Disse space fibrogenesis in alcoholic liver disease. *Hepatology 3*: 559-566.

Nakatsukasa, H., Nagy, P., Evarts, R.P., Hsia, C.C, Marsden, E.,& Thorgeirsson, S.S.(1990): Cellular distribution of transforming growth factor-ß1 and procollagen types I, III, and IV transcripts in carbon tetrachloride-induced rat liver fibrosis. *J. Clin. Invest. 85*: 1833-1843.

Nouchi, T., Tanaka, Y., Tsukada, T., Sato, C.,& Marumo, F.(1991): Appearance of α-smooth muscle-actin-positive cells in hepatic fibrosis. *Liver 11*: 100-105.

Ogawa, K., Suzuki, J.I., Mukai, H.,& Mori, M. (1986): Sequential changes of extracellular matrix and proliferation of Ito cells with enhanced expression of desmin and actin in focal hepatic injury. *Am. J. Pathol. 125*: 611-619.

Pinzani, M., Abboud, H.E.,& Aron, D.C.(1990a): Secretion of insulin-like growth factor-I and binding proteins by rat liver fat-storing cells: regulatory role of platelet-derived growth factor. *Endocrinology 127* :2343-2349.

Pinzani, M., Weber, F.L., Gesualdo, L.,& Abboud,H.E. (1990b): Expression of platelet-derived growth factor (PDGF) in an in vivo model of acute liver inflammation [Abstract]. *Hepatology 12*: 920.

Pinzani, M., Knauss, T.C., Pierce, G.F., Hsieh, P., Kenney, W., Dubyak, G.R.,& Abboud, H.E.(1991): Mitogenic signals for platelet-derived growth factor isoforms in liver fat-storing cells. *Am. J. Physiol. 260*: C485-C491.

Rieder, H., Ramadori, G.,& Meyer zum Büschenfelde, K.H. (1992): Sinusoidal endothelial liver cells in vitro secrete PDGF-like factor(s) stimulating proliferation of cultured liver myofibroblastic cells. In *International Falk Symposium: Molecular and Cell Biology of Liver Fibrogenesis*, Marburg.

Rockey, D.C., Maher, J.J., Gabbiani, G.,& Friedman, S.L. (1991): Interferon gamma (IFN γ) inhibits expression of smooth muscle actin and type I collagen mRNA in rat hepatic lipocytes [Abstract]. *Hepatology 14*: 189A.

Rosenbaum, J., Mavier, P., Preaux, A.M.,& Dhumeaux, D. (1989a): Demonstration of a basic fibroblast growth factor-like molecule in mouse hepatic endothelial cells. *Biochem. Biophys. Res. Commun. 164*: 1099-1104.

Rosenbaum, J., Mavier, P., Preaux, A.M., Lescs, M.C.,& Dhumeaux, D. (1989b): Mouse hepatic endothelial cells in culture secrete a growth inhibitor for hepatic lipocytes and Balb/c 3T3 fibroblasts. *J. Hepatol 9*: 295-300.

Rosenbaum, J., Mallat, A., Preaux, A.M., Mavier, P., Zafrani, E.S.,& Dhumeaux, D.(1991): Effect of polypeptide growth factors on the growth of cultured human hepatic myofibroblast-like cells (transformed Ito cells). In : *Cells of the Hepatic Sinusoid, Vol III*, eds E. Wisse, D.L. Knook, and R.S Mc Cuskey, pp.255-258. Rijswijk : The Kupffer Cell Foundation.

Schmitt-Gräff, A., Krüger, S., Bochard, F., Gabbiani, G.,& Denk, H.(1991): Modulation of alpha smooth muscle actin and desmin expression in perisinusoidal cells of normal and diseased human livers. *Am. J. Pathol. 138*: 1233-1242.

Senoo, H.,& Wake, K. (1985): Suppression of experimental hepatic fibrosis by administration of vitamin A. *Lab. Invest. 52*: 182-194.

Schirmacher, P., Geerts, A., Pietrangelo, A., Dienes, H.P.,& Rogler, C.E. (1991): Hepatocyte growth factor is expressed in fat-storing cells from rat liver, but not in myofibroblast-like cells derived from fat-storing cells [Abstract]. *Hepatology 14*: 95A.

Shiratori, Y., Geerts, A., Ichida, T., Kawase, T.,& Wisse, E. (1986): Kupffer cells from CCl_4-induced fibrotic livers stimulate proliferation of fat-storing cells. *J. Hepatol. 3*: 294-303.

Tanaka, Y., Mak, K.M.,& Lieber, C.S. (1990): Immunohistochemical detection of proliferating lipocytes in regenerating liver. *J. Pathol. 160:* 129-134.

Tanaka, Y., Nouchi, T., Yamane, M., Irie, T., Miyakawa, H., Sato, C.,& Marumo, F.(1991): Phenotypic modulation in lipocytes in experimental liver fibrosis. *J. Pathol. 164*: 273-278.

Widmann, J.J.,& Fashimi, H.D. (1975): Proliferation of mononuclear phagocytes (Kupffer cells) and endothelial cells in regenerating rat liver. *Am. J. Pathol. 80*: 349-366.

Win, K.M., Mallat, A., Charlotte, F., Preaux, A.M., Dumeaux, D., Mavier, P.,& Rosenbaum, J. (1991): Transforming growth factor ß1 (TGFß1) is mitogenic for human Ito cells. Evidence for autocrine involvement of platelet-derived growth factor (PDGF) and basic fibroblast growth factor (bFGF) [Abstract]. *Hepatology 14*: 191A.

Liver Regeneration. Eds D. Bernuau, G. Feldmann. John Libbey Eurotext, Paris © 1992, pp. 49-59.

Cyclin A and liver cell proliferation

Frédérique Zindy[1], Jian Wang[1], Eugénia Lamas[1], Xavier Chenivesse[1], Berthold Henglein[1], Christian Bréchot[1, 2]

[1]INSERM U.75, CHU Necker, 156 rue de Vaugirard, 75742 Paris Cedex 15. [2]Unité d'Hépatologie, Hôpital Laennec, rue de Sèvres, 75007 Paris, France

We have previously reported the identification of hepatitiis B virus (HBV) integration in an intron of cyclin A gene in an early hepatocellular carcinoma and hence the isolation of human cyclin A cDNA.
We have constructed a cDNA library of the original tumor (tumor HEN) and isolated several hybrid HBV-cyclin A cDNAs. These cDNAs have the coding capacity for a HBV-cyclin A fusion protein. In the chimeric protein, the N-terminal of cyclin A, including the signals for signals for cyclin degradation, was deleted and replaced by viral preS2/S sequences while the rest of cyclin A remained intact. HBV integration in the cyclin A gene resulted in the overexpression of hybrid HBV-cyclin A transcripts that code for a stabilized cyclin A.
In addition, we have investigated cyclin A expression in a primary culture of normal rat hepatocytes and during rat liver regeneration after partial hepatectomy. In both cases, cyclin A mRNA and protein accumulate as the cells enter S phase. Moreover we microinjected anti-sense DNA constructs for cyclin A, resulting in effective inhibition of S phase entry.
In conclusion, we showed in this paper an analysis of the expression pattern of cyclin A gene in the original tumor which supports the hypothesis of insertional mutagenesis of HBV, and a study of the role of cyclin A in a normal cell cycle which indicates its involvement in G1/S transition. That cyclin A is involved in S phase may provide new clues as to its potential role in carcinogenesis.

INTRODUCTION :
Cyclins play a major role in the cell cycle regulation. Two classes of cyclins, G1 and M cyclins, have been identified in fission (Booher and Beach, 1988 ; Forsburg and Nurse, 1991) and budding yeast (Hadwiger et al., 1989 ; Nash et al., 1988 ; Ghiara et al., 1991). They cooporate with the gene products of cdc2/cdc28 kinases in driving the cell through G1/S and G2/M boundaries. In higher eukaryotes, several cyclins (cyclins A, B, C, D and E) have been isolated. The cyclin B is a mitotic cyclin, which associates to the p34^{cdc2} protein kinase to initiate mitosis and meiosis (Draetta et

al., 1989 ; Labbé et al., 1989 ; Meijer et al., 1989 ; Gautier et al., 1990). The C, D and E type cyclins seem to act in G1/S boundary since they can rescue G1 cyclin deficient mutants in S. Cerevisiae (Xiong et al., 1991 ; Matsushime et al., 1991 ; Motokura et al., 1991 ; Koff et al., 1991).
Cyclin A can also associate with p34^{cdc2}, but this complex is formed and active in advance of the p34^{cdc2}/cyclin B complex (Swenson et al., 1986 ; Draetta et al., 1989 ; Minshull et al., 1990 ; Pines and Hunter, 1990). However, several lines of evidence suggest that cyclin A may also have a role in the S phase. First, addition of cyclin A to a G1 phase extract was sufficient to initiate SV40 DNA replication in vitro (D'urso et al., 1990) ; second, microinjection of anti-sense cyclin A DNA into cultured cell blocked the initiation of DNA synthesis (see section 2 of this paper) and third, cyclin A associates to a p34^{cdc2} related protein (p33^{cdc2} or CDK2) that functions in S phase (Pines and Hunter, 1990 ; Fang & Newport, 1991 ; Tsai et al., 1991).
We have previously reported the identification of hepatitis B virus (HBV) DNA integration in human cyclin A gene in an early hepatocellular carcinoma (HCC) (Wang et al., 1990). Chronic HBV infection has been associated with the development of HCC by extensive epidemiological studies (Beasley, 1988). There are several mechanisms which account for the role played by HBV in hepatocarcinogenesis. HBV induces cirrhosis, a premalignant state (Chisari et al, 1990). In addition, HBV likely exerts a direct effect on cell transformation by transactivation of the x and truncated PréS2/S viral proteins (Kim et al, 1991) as well by insertional mutagenesis. This latter mechanism has been well illustrated in woodchucks infected with the woodchuck hepatitis virus (WHV) where WHV DNA was found integrated in the C-myc or N-myc gene in 30% of the tumor studied, most of them with an elevated expression of these oncogenes (Fourel et al., 1990). In human, however, there is only one report in which HBV DNA was found to integrate in the gene coding for a retinoic acid receptor β in HCC (Dejean et al., 1986 ; de The et al., 1987).
In the present manuscript we will focus on two implications of our results :
1) a detailed analysis of the expression pattern of cyclin A gene in the original tumor (tumor HEN) which supports the hypothesis of insertional mutagenesis.
2) An analysis of the role of cyclin A in a normal cell cycle which indicates its involvement in G1/S transition.

RESULTS :
1) HBV and cyclin A expression in tumor HEN
In Northern blots of the original tumor HEN, both cyclin A and HBV probes detected the same two polyadenylated transcripts of 2.7 and 1.7 kb, which were nearly the same size as the normal cyclin A transcripts but quite different from that of HBV. These bands were undetectable in the non-tumorous liver of the same patient. A cDNA library was constructed in lambda gt10 with mRNAs from the tumor and hybrid HBV cyclin A transcripts were caracterised.
The genomic structure of the human cyclin A gene has been established in our laboratory (Henglein et al., in preparation). A comparaison with the HBV integration site indicated that the HBV sequences integrated in the first intron of cyclin A gene (Fig. 1). Two representative cDNAs, 1.7 and 2.7 kb respectively, have been completely sequenced. The results indicated that hybrid transcripts

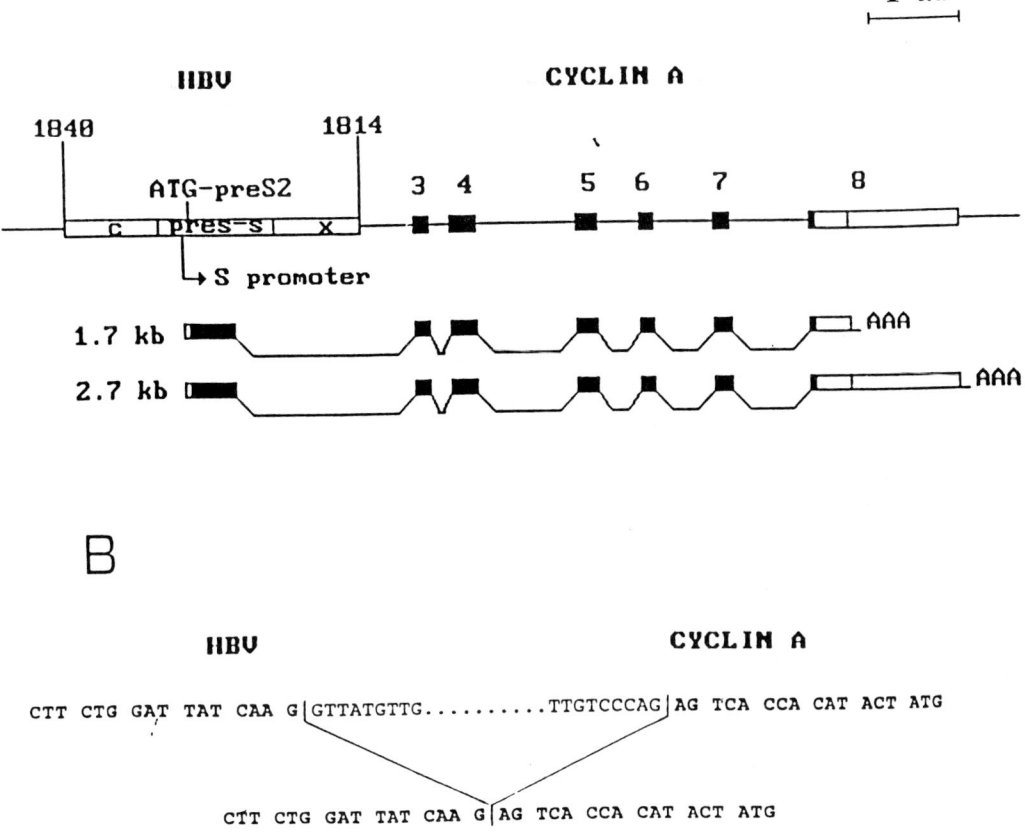

Fig. 1 A : Genomic structure of human cyclin A gene in the HBV integration site (upper) and structure of the hybrid cDNAs (lower). The cyclin A exons are numbered, the black boxs represent the coding sequences and the blanked boxs represent non coding exons, arrow indicate the initiation site of transcription from viral S promoter. The poly (A) tails in the two cDNAs mark the two commonly used polyadenylation sites for normal cyclin A transcription. B : **Sequence of HBV-cyclin A junction in the hybrid cDNAs. The splicing manner is indicated.**

were produced by splicing between HBV and cyclin A sequences, using a cryptic splice donor site in the middle of viral S gene and the normal splice acceptor site of the third exon of cyclin A gene. A primer extension assay, confirmed that the hybrid transcripts were initiated from the viral Pre S2/S promoter (data not shown).
Sequence analysis showed that the HBV open reading frame was fused to that of the cyclin A in the hybrid cDNAs which code for an HBV-cyclin A fusion protein of 430 amino acids. In the chimeric protein, the N-terminal 152 amino acids of cyclin A were reimplaced by 150 amino acids from the viral PreS2 and a part of S regions whereas the

C-terminal two third of cyclin A, including the cyclin box, remained intact (Fig. 1). In vitro translation of the hybrid cDNA produced a 54 KD protein (slightly smaller than normal cyclin A). The N-terminal domain of cyclin A contains the signals for its degradation by the ubiquitin pathway, (Glotzer et al., 1991). An in vitro degradation assay recently indicated that the deletion of the N-terminal of cyclin A has indeed stabilized cyclin A (data not shown).

2) Cyclin A is required in S phase in normal epithelial cells.

Until now, the investigations on cyclins have been performed either in invertebrates or in transformed mammalian cells. Therefore, we chose to investigate cyclin A expression in normal epithelial cells. With this purpose, we have studied cyclin A mRNA and protein in primary culture of rat hepatocytes and in rat liver regeneration. This approach was associated to experiments based on microinjecting an anti-sense cyclin A cDNA.

In vitro cultured hepatocytes can be maintained for 8 days in serum-free medium supplemented with dexamethasone and insulin (referred to as untreated hepatocytes). Alternatively, culturing cells in serum-free medium supplemented with insulin, pyruvate and epidermal growth factor (EGF) (referred to as treated hepatocytes), stimulates DNA synthesis in most hepatocytes (around 80%), with a maximum at day 3 of culture (Mc Gowan, 1986). Using these experimental conditions, we established primary rat hepatocytes culture confirming that maximum DNA synthesis, shown by ^{3}H-thymidine incorporation, occured on day 3 in treated hepatocytes (fig. 2A). When the hepatocytes were untreated, DNA synthesis was barely detectable. Initial experiments used Northern analysis of cyclin A mRNAs. Cyclin A mRNA was not detected in untreated hepatocytes (fig. 2B). In contrast, in treated hepatocytes, the accumulation of cyclin A mRNA increased to a maximum at day 2-4 and then decreased (fig. 2B). This accumulation of transcripts coincided with maximal ^{3}H-thymidine incorporation. To determine if these transcripts were effectively related to protein expression, we also analyzed total cellular protein from cultured hepatocytes by means of immunoblotting with affinity purified polyclonal antibodies raised against human cyclin A. In primary culture, cyclin A protein was detectable from day 2 to day 5 with a maximum at day 3 in treated hepatocytes (i.e. at the time of DNA synthesis) (fig. 2C). Furthermore, we analyzed the localization of cyclin A in cultured hepatocytes. The staining of cyclin A was preferentially localized into the nucleus. At day 3 of culture, high amount of cells were labelled for cyclin A whereas at day 1 of culture, only few cells were stained (data not shown).

To determine if this observation also true in-vivo, the expression of cyclin A was analysed in regenerating liver at various times after partial hepatectomy (PH). Indeed, PH partially synchronizes the hepatocytes proliferative phase (30-40%) during the first mitosis. The growth process includes a distinct prereplicative phase of hypertrophy which lasts for 12-16 hrs after PH and a replicative phase in which hepatocytes undergo DNA replication (peak et 24 hrs) and then division (peak at 30 hrs) (Bucher and Malt, 1971 ; Grisham, 1962).

Therefore, we analyzed liver samples obtained at 16 to 32 hrs after PH. After 32 hrs, further points were not analyzed due to the loss of cellular synchronisation. ^{3}H-thymidine incorporation was detected with a maximum at 24 hrs after PH (fig. 3A). Northern blot analysis revealed cyclin A mRNA at a very low level before and 16 hrs after

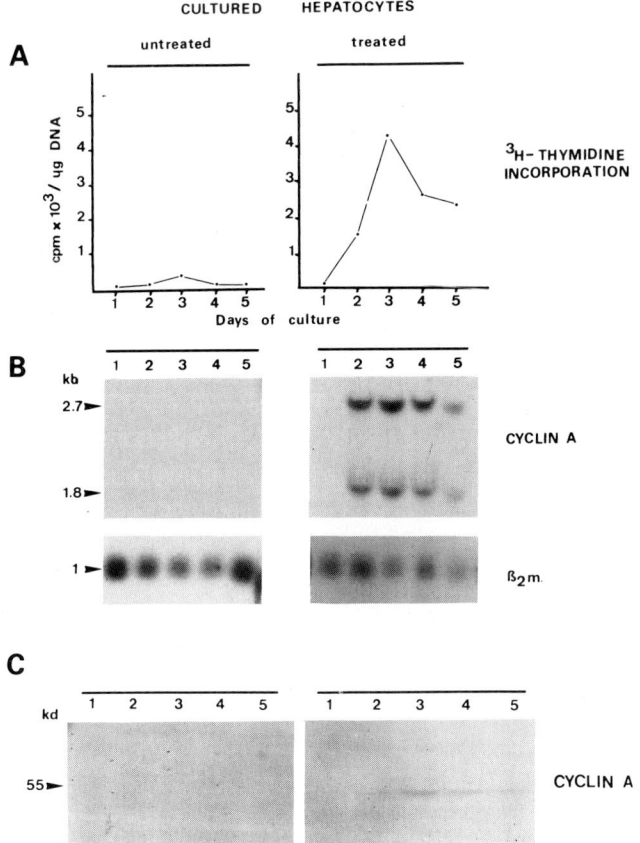

Fig. 2 : **Cyclin A expression and ^{3}H-Thymidine incorporation in cultured hepatocytes.** Hepatocytes were isolated from 2-month-old male Wistar rats and cultured in serum-free medium supplemented with dexamethasone (1μM) and insulin (200nUI/ml) (untreated hepatocytes) or in serum-free medium supplemented with insulin (20 m UI/ml), pyruvate (20 mM) and epidermal growth factor (50ng/ml) (treated hepatocytes). Hepatocytes untreated or treated by growth factors were harversted at the indicated times. ^{3}H-thymidine incorporation was measured (A), cyclin A mRNAs were analyzed by Northern blot normalized relative to B2 microglobulin mRNAs (B2m.) (B), and cyclin A protein was analyzed by Western blot (C).

PH (fig. 3B). Cyclin A mRNA accumulation increased at 20 hrs with a maximum level from 24 hrs to 32 hrs after PH corresponding respectively to the period in which maximal DNA synthesis and mitosis take place. Cyclin A protein was not detected before or 16 hrs after PH (fig. 3C) ; its level was maintained from 24-26 hrs (time of DNA synthesis) to 32 hrs (time of mitosis).

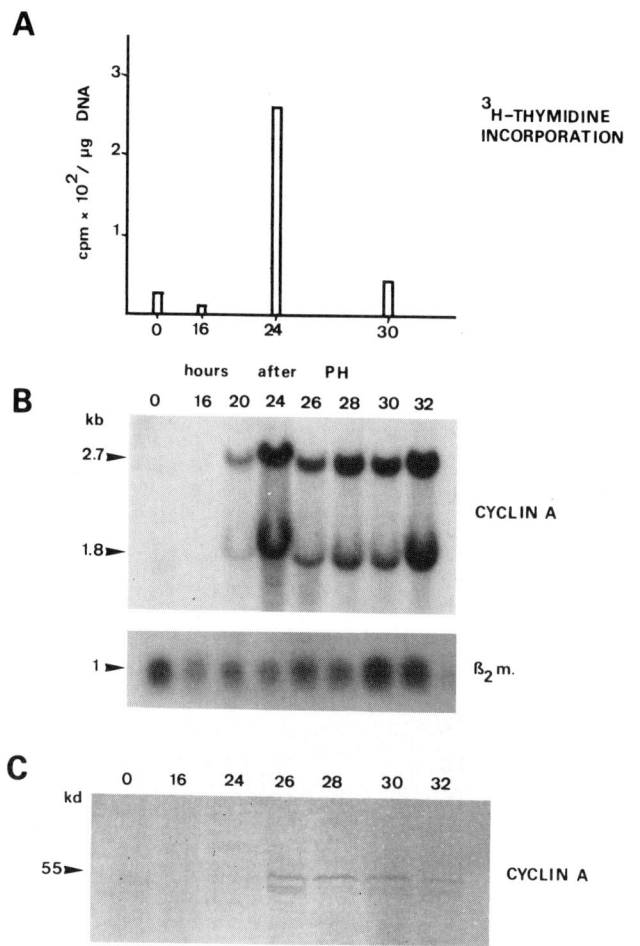

Fig. 3 : cyclin A expression and ^{3}H-thymidine incorporation in regenerating liver after partial hepatectomy. Male Wistar rats were subjected to 70% partial hepatectomy and liver was removed at the indicated times after hepatectomy. ^{3}H-thymidine incorporation was measured (A), cyclin A mRNAs were analyzed by Northern blot normalized relative to B2 microglobulin (B2m.) (B), and cyclin A protein was analyzed by Western blot.

To examine further the effects of changes in cyclin A mRNA and protein levels, we investigated the consequences on S phase transit of artificially inhibiting cyclin A synthesis. We inhibited cyclin A synthesis through microinjection of plasmid constructs encoding anti-sense human cyclin A cDNA under the control of SV40 promoter-enhancer element. At various times after plating, cultured rat hepatocytes stimulated by growth factors were microinjected with the anti-sense cyclin A construct, a sense cyclin A construct or an anti-sense human cyclin B cDNA under the control of an SV40 promotor-enhancer element. The effects of injection were assessed by following the incorporation of 5-bromo-deoxyuridine (5-Br-DU) (i.e. S-phase transit). Injected cells were relocated by inclusion of a non-specific antibody in the injection solutions which was subsequently stained after immunofluorescence with anti-5-Br-DU. Cells were injected 2-3 days after plating and labelled from injection until the end of day 4. Each microinjection experiment was performed three times, involving the injection of 30 to 40 cells every time. Under normal conditions, treated hepatocytes synthetized DNA between the end of day 2 and day 5 (as controlled by ^{3}H-thymidine and 5-Br-DU incorporation). The pattern of 5-Br-DU staining was similar in cells injected with the sense cyclin A construct (data not shown) and in cells injected with the anti-sense cyclin B construct (fig. 4 pannels A and B) which showed between 50 to 85% of DNA synthesis, a level similar to that achieved in the surrounding non injected cells. In contrast, cells injected with the anti-sense cyclin A construct (fig. 4 pannels C-F, and table 1), showed no evidence of DNA synthesis if injected during day 2 (C and D) or day 3 (E and F) ; we detected no evidence of nuclear staining for cyclin A in injected cells (data not shown). Surrounding uninjected cells proceeded normally to transit S-phase. This effect was observed in all the cells injected with the anti-sense constructs from the end of day 2 until day 3.

DISCUSSION :
In this paper, we have both analyzed the HBV and cyclin A expression in the tumor HEN and further caracterized the role of cyclin A in a normal cell cycle.
Concerning the tumor HEN, we have provided strong evidence for a role of HBV in a step of liver cell transformation by insertional mutagenesis. Indeed we showed an increased level of hybrid transcripts HBV-cyclin A, potentially coding for a stabilized chimeric protein. There are several possibilities to account for its effect on the cell phenotype. Loss of the degradation signals in the N-terminal part of the cyclin A, together with initiation from the Pre S2/S viral promoter, may lead to an increased and constitutive synthesis of cyclin A. In addition it is also plausible that the membranous PreS2/S protein may markedly change the localization in the cell of the protein. Finally the viral sequences at the N-terminal part include a truncated form of PreS/S which may have retained a transactivating effect on cellular oncogenes (Kekule et al., 1990 ; Caselman et al., 1990). These different possibilities are being explored through in vitro transfection of cell cultures and in vivo experiments on transgenic mice.
In order to clarify the involvement of cyclin A in carcinogenesis, we have also adressed the issue of its potential role in the G1/S phase of the cell cycle. The present study provides two lines of evidence for the requirement of cyclin A for the cell to proceed to S phase. First, cyclin A mRNA and protein are accumulated as the cells enter S phase in hepatocytes in-vitro and in-vivo. Secondly, the microinjection of an anti-sense cyclin A cDNA inhibited DNA synthesis in cultured normal epithelial cells. The involvememt of cyclin A in the S phase was further supported by the specific inhibition of DNA synthesis following the microinjection of an anti-sense cyclin A while an anti-sense cyclin B cDNA did not inhibit DNA synthesis. Therefore, our observation, based on normal epithelial cells analyzed in-vitro and in-vivo, does imply that cyclin A is not only a mitotic cyclin but also acts at S phase. This finding is also

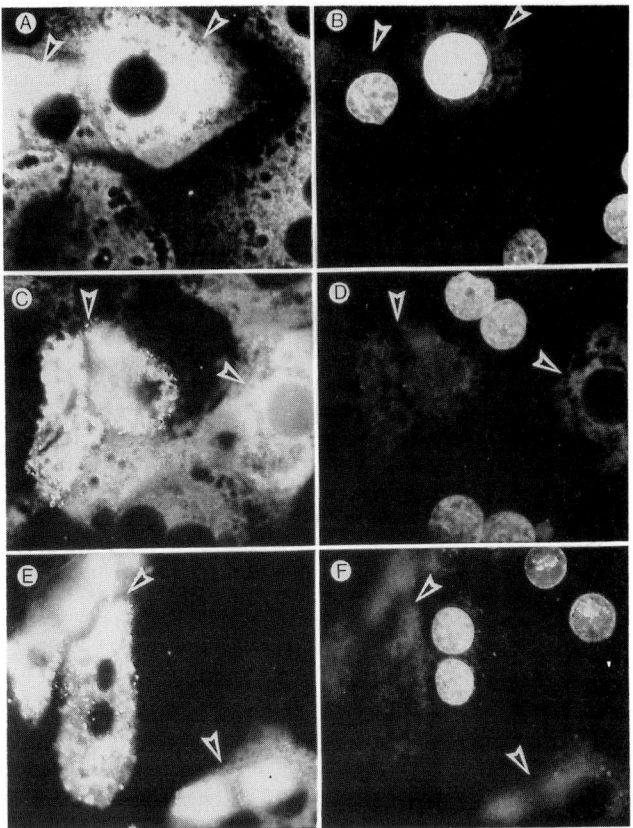

Fig. 4 : **effect on DNA synthesis in cultured hepatocytes of overexpression of anti-sense cyclin constructs.** To examine the involvement of cyclin A in S phase transit in cultured hepatocytes, cells stimulated by growth factors (day 0) were microinjected with either anti-sense human cyclin A or B cDNA under transcriptional regulation of a SV40 enhancer element. Immediately afterwards, cells were incubated in the presence of 5-Br-DU.
Cells were stained for the distribution of 5-Br-DU (panels B, D, F) and subsequently for the non-specific anti-serum co-injected with the DNA (panels A, C, E). Shown are cells injected on the second day of culture (panels A-D) and cells injected on the third day of culture (panels E and F). Cells were microinjected with either an anti-sense cyclin B (panels A-B), or anti-sense cyclin A (panels C-F) cDNA constructs. Arrowed are the injected cells.

consistent with recent in-vitro reports based on cell-free replication of simian virus 40 DNA (D'Urso et al, 1990). In view of our present observation on the role of cyclin A in S phase, it is interesting to note that cyclin A has been recently shown to associate to E_2F transcription factor in S phase (Mudryj et al,

1991), and to be included in a complex containing the retinoblastinoma protein and the DRTF1 transcription factor (related to E2F) (Bandara et al, 1991). It is therefore possible that cyclin A plays a role in regulation of transcription. Our result also raises the question as to the nature of cdc2 protein kinase which associates to cyclin A. Cyclin A has been shown to complex both to $p34^{cdc2}$ as well as to a $p33^{cdc2}$ (Pines and Hunter, 1990), recently referred to as CDCK2 (Tsai et al., 1991).
Therefore, this study might be important with regard to the potential involvement of cyclin A in cell transformation. Indeed, cyclin A has been shown to associate with the E1A protein of adenovirus in infected cells (Giordano et al 1983). In addition, hepatitis B virus DNA has integrated into the cyclin A gene in a human primary liver cancer. That cyclin A is involved in S phase may provide new clues as to its potential role in carcinogenesis.

REFERENCES

Bandara, L.R. & La Thangue, N.B. (1991) : Cyclin A and the retinoblastoma gene product complex with a common transcription factor. Nature 351, 494-497.
Beasley, R.P. (1988) : Hepatitis B virus : the major etiology of hepatocellular carcinoma. Cancer Res. 61, 1942-1956.
Booher, R., and Beach, D. (1988) : Involvement of cdc13+ in mitotic control in Schizosacchromyces pombe : possible interaction of the gene product with microtubules. EMBO J. 7, 2321-2327.
Bucher, N.L.R. & Malt, R.A. (1971) : Regeneration of liver and kidney. Little, Brown & Co, New-York, 1-278.
Caselman, W.H., Meyer, M., Kekule, A.S., Lauer, U., Hofscheneider, P.H. & Koshy, R. (1990) : A trans-activator function is generated by integration of hepatitis B virus preS/S sequences in human hepatocellular carcinoma DNA. Proc. Natl. Acad. Sci. USA 87, 2970-2974.
Chisari, F.V., Klopchin, K., Moriyama, T., Pasquinelli, C., Dunsford, H.A., Sell, S. Pinkert, C.A., Brinster, R.L. & Palmer, R.D. 1990 : Molecular pathogenesis of hepatocellular carcinoma in hepatitis B virus transgenic mice. Cell 59, 1145-1156.
Dejean, A., Bougueleret, L., Grzeschik, K.H., & Tiollais, P. (1986) : Hepatitis B virus DNA integration in a sequence homologous to v-erb-A and steroid receptor gene in a hepatocellular carcinoma. Nature 322, 70-72.
Draetta, G. Luca, F., Westendorf, J., Brizuela, L., Ruderman, J. & Beach, D. (1989) : cdc2 protein kinase is complexed with both cyclin A and B : evidence for proteolytic inactivation of MPF. Cell 56, 829-838.
Fang, F. & Newport, J.W. (1991) : Evidence that the G1-S and G2-M transitions are controlled by differnt cdc2 proteins in higher eukaryotes. Cell, 66, 731-742.
Forsburg, S.L., and Nurse, P. (1991) : Identification of a G1-type cyclin puc1+ in the fission yeast Schizosaccharomyces pombe. Nature 351, 245-248.
Fourel, G., Trepo, C., Bougueleret, L., Henglein, B., Ponzetto, A., Tiollais, P. & Buendia, M.A. (1990) : Frequent activation of N-myc genes by hepadnavirus insertion in

woodchuck liver tumours. Nature 347, 294-298.
Gautier, J., Minshull, J. Lohka, M., Glotzer, M., Hunt, & Maller, J.L. (1990) : Cyclin is a compoment of maturing-promoting -factor from Xenopus. Cell 60, 487-494.
Ghiara, J.B., Richardson, H.E., Sugimoto, K., Henze, M., Lew, D.J., Wittenberg, C. & Reed, S.I. (1991) : A cyclin B homolog in S. cerevisiae : chronic activation of the cdc28 protein kinase prevents exit from mitosis. Cell 65, 163-174.
Giordanno, A., Whyte, P., Harlow, Ed., Franza, B.R., Beach, D., Draetta, G. (1989) : A 60 kd cdc2-associated polypeptide complexes with the E1A proteins in adenovirus-infected cells. Cell 58, 981-990.
Glotzer, M., Murray, A.W. & Kirschner, M.W. (1991) : Cyclin is degraded by the ubiquitin pathway. Nature 349, 132-137.
Grisham, J.W., (1962) : A morphologic study of deoxyribonucleic acid synthesis and cell proliferation in regenerating rat liver ; autoradiography with Thymidine-^{3}H. Cancer Res. 22, 842-849.
Hadwiger, J.A., Wittenberg, C., Richardson, H.E., de Barros Lopes, M. & Reed, S.I. (1989) :A family of cyclin homologs that control the G1 phase in yeast. Proc. Natl. Acad. Sci. USA 86, 6255-6259.
Kekulé, A.S., Lauer, U., Meyer, M., Caselman, W.H., Hofschneider, P.H. & Koshy, R. (1990) : The preS2/S region of integrated hepatitis B virus encodes a transcriptionnal transactivator. Nature 343, 457-460.
Kim, C.M., Koike, K., Saito, I., Miyamura, T. & Jay, G. (1991) : HBx gene of hepatitis B virus induces liver cancer in transgenic mice. Nature 351, 317-320.
Koff, A., Cross, A., Fisher, A., Schuma, J., Le Guellec, K., Philippe, M. & Roberts, J.M. (1991) : Human cyclin E, a new cyclin that interacts with two members of the cdc2 gene family. Cell 66, 1217-1228.
Labbé, J.C., Capony, J.P., Caput, D., Cavadore, J.C., Derancourt, J., Kaghad, M., Lelias, J.M., Picard, A. & Dorée, M. (1989) : MPF from starfish oocytes at first meiotic metaphase is a heterodimer containing one molecule of cdc2 and one molecule of cyclin B. EMBO J. 8, 3053-3058.
Matsushime, H., Roussel, M.F., Ashum, R.A. & Sherr, C.J. (1991) : Colony-stimulating factor 1 regulates novel cyclins during the G1 phase of the cell cycle. Cell 65, 701-713.
Meijer, L., Arion, D., Golsteyn, R., Pines, J., Brizuela, L., Hunt, T. & Beach, D. (1989) :Cyclin is a compoment of the sea urchin egg M-phase specific histone H1 kinase. EMBO J. 8, 2275-2282.
Mc Gowan, J.A. (1986) : prolifération des hépatocytes en culture Research in... Isolated and cultured hepatocytes. INSERM/John Libbey Eurotext, 13-40.
Minshull, J., Golsteyn, R., Hill, C.S. & Hunt T. (1990) :The A- and B-type cyclin associated cdc2 kinase in Xenopus turn on and off at different times in the cell cycle. Embo J. 9, 2865-2875.
Motokura, T., Bloom, T., Kim, H.G., Juppner, H., Ruderman, J.V., Kronenberg, H.M. & Arnold, A. (1991) : A novel cyclin encoded by a bcl1-linked candidate oncogene. Nature 350, 512-515.
Nash, R., Tokiwa, G., Anand, S., Erickson, K. & Futcher, A.B. (1988) : The WHI1+ gene of Saccharomyces cerevisiae tethers

cell division to cell size and is a cyclin homolog. EMBO J. 7, 4335-4346.
Pines, J., & Hunter, T. (1990) : Human cyclin A is adenovirus E1A-associated protein p60 and behaves differently from cyclin B. Nature 346, 760-763.
Swenson, K.I., Farell, K.M. & Ruderman, J.V. (1986) : The clam embryo protein cyclin A induces entry into M phase and resumption of meiosis in Xenopus oocytes. Cell 47, 861-870.
de Thé, H., Marchio, A., Tiollais, P. & Dejean, A. (1987) : A novel steroid thyroid hormone receptor-related gene inappropriately expressed in human hepatocellular carcinoma. Nature 330, 667-670.
Tsai, L.H., Harlow, E. & Meyerson, M. (1991) : Isolation of the cdk2 gene that encodes the cyclin A- and adenovirus E1A-associated p33 kinase. Nature 353, 174-177.
D'Urso, G., Marraciano, R.L., Marchak, D.K., & Roberts, J.M. (1990) : Cell cycle control of DNA replication by a homologue from human cells of the $p34^{cdc2}$ protein kinase. Science 250, 786-791.
Wang, J., Chenivesse, X., Henglein, B., Bréchot, C. (1990) : Hepatitis B virus integration in a cyclin A gene in a hepatocellular carcinoma. Nature 343, 555-557.
Xiong, Y., Connolly, T., Futcher, B. & Beach, D. (1991) : Human D-type cyclin. Cell 65, 691-699.

Liver Regeneration. Eds D. Bernuau, G. Feldmann. John Libbey Eurotext, Paris © 1992, pp. 61-69.

Cell cycle progression of adult rat hepatocytes *in vitro*

Pascal Loyer, Denise Glaise, Laurent Meijer*, Christiane Guguen-Guillouzo

*INSERM U.49, Hôpital Pontchaillou, Rennes and *CNRS, Station Biologique, Roscoff, France*

Abstract

In primary culture, adult hepatocytes can be stimulated by insulin, Epidermal Growth Factor (EGF) and pyruvate to undergo DNA synthesis. The aim of this work was to use this in vitro model: 1) to define the different phases of the cell cycle in growing normal hepatocytes; 2) to analyze in parallel the expression of p34cdc2 protein, its associated Histone H1 kinase activity (H1K) and the sequence of proto-oncogene activation; 3) to compare the data to those obtained *in vivo* during liver regeneration after partial hepatectomy (PHT). In vitro, the S phase, characterized by ^{3}H-thymidine-uptake, started 48 hours (hr) after cell seeding. Maximal DNA synthesis takes place at 84 hr whereas the maximum of mitotic figures was obtained at around 96 hr. *In vivo*, DNA synthesis started at 18 hr after PHT, reached a maximum at 24 hr, and then gradually decreased, according to results previously reported (Grisham, 1962; Fabrikant, 1968). In both *in vivo* and *in vitro* systems, when extracts were made throughout the cell cycle, the p34cdc2 protein was detected only after G1/S transition and increased thereafter, reaching a maximum during G2 and M phases. No p34cdc2 protein was detected during G1 phase. In addition, quantification of the tyrosine phosphorylated form of p34cdc2 protein showed an accumulation during the S phase followed by a gradual disappearance, indicating the progression through the G2 and towards the M phase. This finding was confirmed by activation of H1K during the same period. *In vivo*, a sequential activation of proto-oncogenes, including c-fos, c-myc, p53, the jun and the ras families, has been reported to parallel hepatocyte growth activity during liver regeneration after two-third hepatectomy. This activation has been found *in vitro*, and further analyzed in relation with the cell cycle progression. A transient increase of c-fos and c-jun transcripts was observed during liver tissue disruption indicating an early transition from G0 to G1 phase in isolated cells. Then, c-myc and jun B were expressed at a high level up to the cell entrance in S phase (48 hr) while p53 and jun D occurred during the G1 phase and remained overexpressed all along the cell cycle. C-Ki-ras was slightly expressed during G1 phase and strongly increased at the G1/S transition. These results: 1) show that p34cdc2 plays a major role in the G2/M transition, but not in the G1/S transition, in rat hepatocytes; 2) indicate that activation of some proto-oncogenes was related to G0/G1 transition while others were related to G1 and G1/S phases. They demonstrate that EGF/pyruvate-stimulated hepatocyte culture is a suitable system to study mechanisms of cell cycle progression.

Introduction

In normal liver, cells divide at a very low rate (<< 1% daily) and at the adult stage this tissue keeps the possibility to regenerate after partial mass loss (Higgins & Anderson, 1931). PHT triggers the proliferation of liver cells which undergo DNA synthesis and division up to mass tissue recovery within few days (Fabrikant, 1968; Grisham, 1962). This regenerative process can be mimicked *in vitro* and advantageously used to further analyze the mechanisms which control the cell cycle progression. Different *in vitro* models have been described that allow hepatocyte DNA synthesis (**table 1**, McGowan, 1986). Among them, addition of a mixture of insulin, Epidermal Growth Factor (EGF) and pyruvate was reported as the most efficient supplied medium (EGF/pyr) inducing an intense DNA replicative phase. However, unexpectedly only few mitotic figures were reported (Friedman et al., 1981; Hasegawa et al., 1982; Richman et al., 1976), and the completion of the cell cycle in the whole population remained questionable.

Table 1 :Major humoral growth stimulating factors of adult hepatocytes.

Mitogenic factors	Co-mitogenic factors
EGF	Norepinephrin
TGF	Vasopressin
HBGF-I or FGF	Oestrogens
Hepatopoietin A or HGF	Angiotensin I and II
PDGF	Insulin
	Glucagon

The p34cdc2 gene has been described to encode a cell cycle kinase protein considered as a master effector which controls the restriction points (G1/S and G2/M transitions) in fission yeast Schizosaccharomyces pombe cell cycle (Nurse & Bissett, 1981; Piggott et al, 1982). More recently, cdc2 has also been shown to play a crucial role in G2/M transition in a large range of proliferating eukaryotic cells (Arion et al, 1988; Draetta et al, 1988; Lee et al, 1988). However, in mammals its role in G1/S transition is still yet discussed. Indeed, data from different transformed cell lines seemed to confirm a p34cdc2 control of G1/S transition while others suggested that G1/S and G2/M transitions may be controlled by distinct cell cycle kinases (Elledge et Spottswood, 1991; Fang et Newport, 1991; Paris et al., 1991). We have devised experiments using both the *in vitro* EGF/pyr-stimulated hepatocytes and *in vivo* regenerating liver to investigate the role of p34cdc2 in normal proliferating cells.

Numerous studies have described a sequential proto-oncogene activation after PHT (Corral et al, 1985; Morello et al, 1990; Sobczack et al, 1989; Thompson et al, 1986), thereby underlying for each of them, distinct roles in the cell cycle progression (**fig 1**). However, this sequential activation of proto-oncogenes remained widely controversial when compared to other proliferating cell systems (Thompson et al., 1985). Only few reports described proto-oncogene expression in hepatocyte primary cultures. We have previously demonstrated a transient overexpression of c-fos after tissue disruption of rat liver, and a maintenance of c-myc in long-term culture of normal adult rat hepatocytes (Etienne et al, 1988). Sawada (1989) also showed activation of c-myc in short-term cultured hepatocytes treated or not with EGF and suggested that hepatocytes might progress from G0 to G1 phase even in the absence of DNA synthesis. This hypothesis was confirmed by Ikeda et al. (1989).

In this work, we have established the sequence of proto-oncogene activation in cultured dividing hepatocytes with respect to cell cycle progression and p34cdc2 expression.

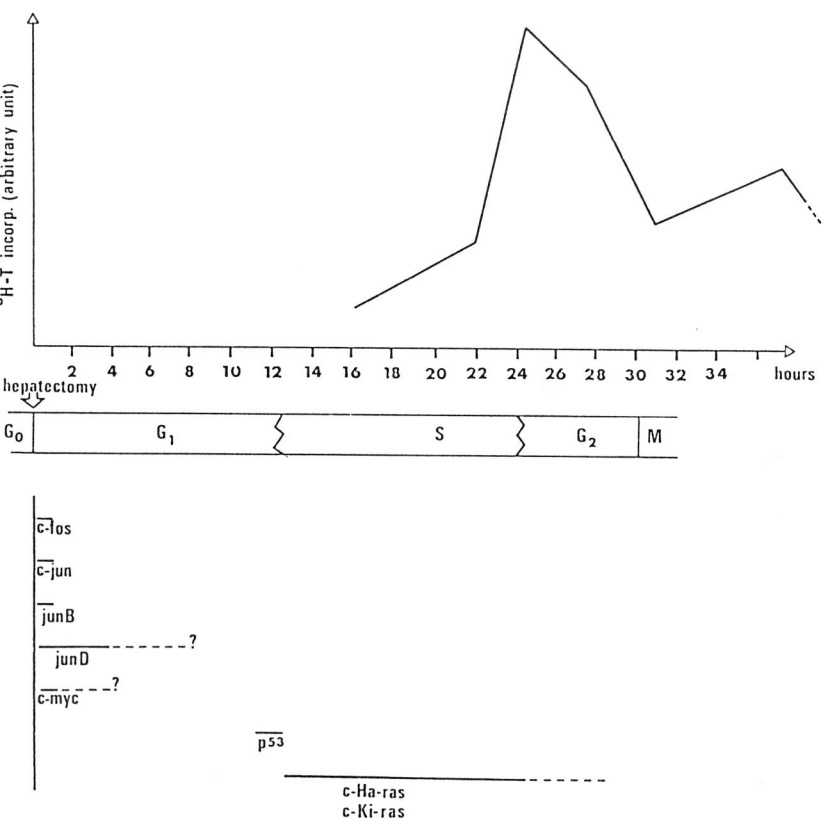

Figure 1: Schematic representation of the sequential proto-oncogene activation during rat liver regeneration.

Results

Comparable cell cycle of normal adult hepatocytes when stimulated to proliferate either *in vitro* or in *in vivo* regenerating liver.

In vitro, when the basal medium was added with insulin (5µg/ml) and glucocorticoids (0.1µM; hydrocortisone) only, no ^{3}H-thymidine incorporation was detectable during the first 36 hours of culture, and only very low level of DNA synthesis could be observed from 2 to 6 days of culture. In contrast, when both EGF (50 ng/ml) and pyruvate (20mM) were added to the basal medium together with insulin and glucocorticoids, DNA synthesis was increased at least 10-fold (**fig 2**). Interestingly, no DNA synthesis occurred before 48 hr of culture, indicating a G1 phase of 48 hr. The S phase started 48 hr after cell seeding and maximum DNA synthesis was found at about 84 hr. Numerous typical mitotic figures demonstrated the high rate of divisions (**fig 3**).

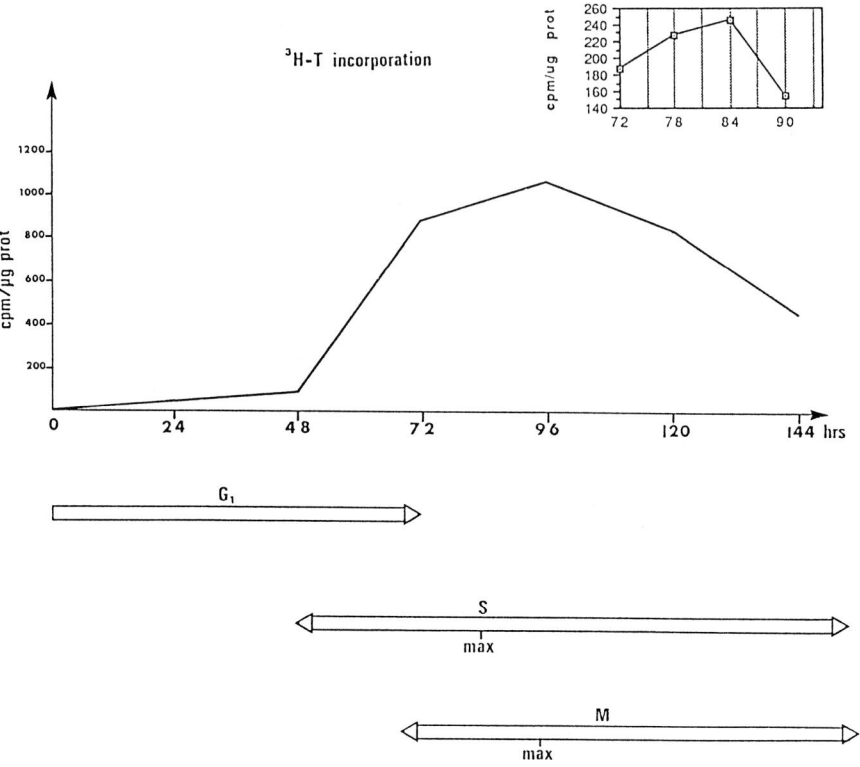

Figure 2: ^{3}H-Thymidine incorporation in EGF-pyr stimulated hepatocytes and schematic representation of G1, S and M phases.

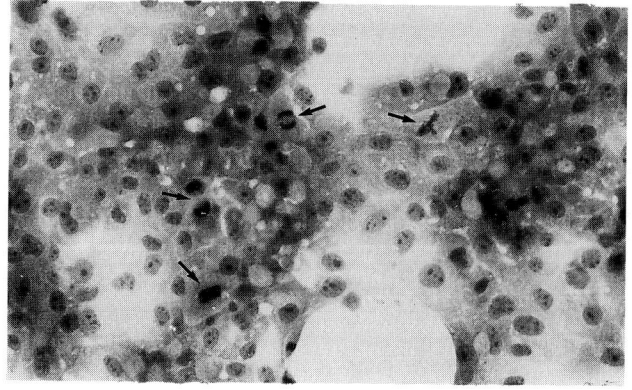

Figure 3: Evidence of mitotic activity in 4-day old primary cultures of normal adult rat hepatocytes. Cells were fixed and stained by May-Grunwald and Giemsa. Mitotic figures (↑) can be observed (x500).

Mitotic index was established by counting the cells blocked in M phase following colcemid treatment. It was low (< 1/1000) during the first 48 hr after plating, increased to 10 % at 72hr and reached a maximum (50%) at about 96hr. Thereafter DNA synthesis and mitotic rate decreased sharply, corresponding to less than 5% of mitotic cells per day. Taken together, these results show that EGF/pyr induced most hepatocytes to enter the G1 and S phases in a synchronized manner and to progress through one complete cell cycle. This makes stimulated hepatocyte primary culture a very appropriate model for analyzing the different events which control progression through the different phases.

In vivo, liver regeneration follows a biphasic response as previously reported (Grisham, 1962; Fabrikant, 1968; Thompson & al., 1985; Sobczak and Duguet, 1986). During the first mitotic round, only the hepatocytes are involved in DNA replication (peak 24 hr) and mitotic activity (peak 30 hr). The second mitotic round, which is less synchronous, occurs about 24 hr later, and includes both hepatocytes and non parenchymal cells. Mitotic figures can still be observed during the next days, but mitotic index becomes very low, and after 6-7 days regenerating liver process is achieved. In order to confirm this temporal pattern, we have performed a time course of ^{3}H-Thymidine incorporation in liver after PHT. As expected, no DNA synthesis was observed before 16-18 hr after PHT, the peak of replication occurred at 24 hr after PHT, followed by a gradual decrease. Then, our results are completely the same as those previously reported. For the following experiments, we have focussed our attention on the first mitotic wave (PHT to 36 hr after PHT) in which a large number of hepatocytes divide synchronously.

p34cdc2 protein expression and Histone H1 kinase activity during the cell cycle of normal hepatocytes.

We have defined p34cdc2 expression through the cell cycle and determined its role in G1/S and G2/M transitions by using both the *in vivo* regenerating and *in vitro* EGF/pyr systems of normal dividing hepatocytes (**fig 4**).

a) p34cdc2 protein expression

Analyses were performed on both mRNA and protein molecules. *In vitro*, by northern blot analysis we failed to detect p34cdc2 mRNA during the first 36 hr after plating. A faint band was detected after 48 hr of culture; its expression gradually increased up to a maximum between 72-84 hr and decreased thereafter. In addition, p34cdc2 protein was detected by western blot. It was weakly expressed 54 hr after plating, increased with time until 84 hr, remained stable, and then drastically decreased after 120 hr of culture (**fig 4**).

In regenerating liver, by northern-blot analysis we have never detected p34cdc2 mRNA before 18 hr. Its relative amount increased from 18 to 24 hr and decreased thereafter but did not completely disappear. P34cdc2 protein was found by western-blotting (by using a specific antibody directed against C-terminal-part of p34cdc2) from 18 to 36 hr after PHT, corresponding to S, G2 and M phases. p34cdc2 appeared as a faint band at 18 hr; its relative level dramatically increased up to 24 hr, remained stable until 28 hr and increased again until its maximum at 32 hr. p34cdc2 decreased only after 36 hr. Interestingly, a double band was observed between 22 to 28 hr, suggesting two different p34cdc2 phosphorylated forms. Thus, this protein appeared to be synthetized during S and G2 phases, as in cultured hepatocytes.

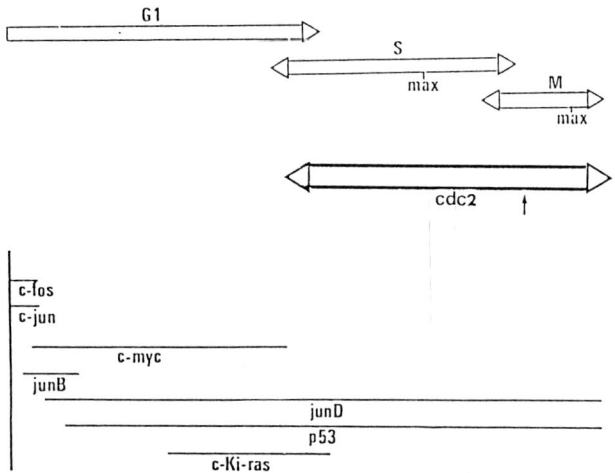

Figure 4: Schematic representation of the sequential cdc2 and proto-oncogene activation during cell cycle of normal adult rat hepatocytes in both in vivo and in vitro systems. (†) indicates the time at which cdc2 is maximally expressed.

b) <u>Histone H1 kinase activity</u>

The cascade of phosphorylation/dephosphorylation and kinase activity of purified cdc2-related kinases was followed along the cell cycle in both *in vitro* and *in vivo* systems. Quantitation of the tyrosine phosphorylated form of p34cdc2 which is an inactive form of this protein kinase, showed no expression during G1 phase, an accumulation during S phase followed by a decrease, in the cell cycle progression towards the G2 and M phases. Moreover, the p34cdc2 kinase activity (using histone H1 as substrat) was found high at G2/M transition. However a phosphorylation of histone H1 was also detected during S phase. This activity might be related to the active dephosphorylated form of p34cdc2 and/or to another cdc2-related kinase.

Proto-oncogene activation during the cell cycle of cultured hepatocytes.

In vivo, an overexpression of some proto-oncogenes in liver after partial hepatectomy, has been shown (Corral et al., 1985 ; Thompson et al., 1986 ; Sobczack et al., 1989; Morello et al., 1990). In order to progress in the understanding of the role of proto-oncogenes in the cell cycle, we have analyzed the level expression of 7 of them: c-fos, c-myc, p53, c-Ki-ras and jun family. All these proto-oncogenes were induced in the EGF/pyr-stimulated hepatocyte model (**Fig. 4**). c-fos and c-jun overexpression took place very early during cell isolation, indicating that hepatocytes entered G1 phase following tissue disruption. In contrast, jun D, jun B and c-myc expression increased in isolated cells and reached a maximum 6 hr after cell plating. p53 was weakly expressed in freshly isolated cells, slightly increased 6 hr after plating and was highly expressed at 24 hr. Thereafter, jun B and c-myc decreased whereas jun D and p53 were maintained all along the cell cycle, including the S and M phases. We have confirmed the G1-related expression of c-myc by using sodium butyrate which blocks the cells in early G1 phase. Treated hepatocytes exhibited a high level of c-myc mRNA all along the culture time. For c-Ki-ras, a faint band was detected in whole liver and in freshly isolated hepatocytes. It was slightly enhanced at 6 and 24 hr, reached a maximum at 48 hr and declined thereafter.

Conclusion.

We have established for both *in vitro* and *in vivo* proliferating hepatocyte systems the p34cdc2 expression and kinase activity and proto-oncogene activation with respect to the different phases of the cell cycle. By these experiments, we confirm that *in vitro*, normal rat hepatocytes are able to undergo a complete and synchronous cell cycle with mechanisms of phosphorylation/dephosphorylation, kinase activation and proto-oncogene expression, similar to the *in vivo* situation. However, an important discrepancy has been observed in the length of the cell cycle between the two models. Indeed, the cell cycle lasts 96 hr *in vitro* while it does not exceed 32 hr *in vivo*. This very long cell cycle *in vitro*, probably reflecting the cell adaptation to culture environment, appears to be a unique situation to further analyze specific cellular and molecular aspects of regulation which controls each cell cycle phase.
In addition, our data provide strong evidence for a major role of p34cdc2 during the G2/M transition, but not during the G1/S transition. Further experiments should be devised to define the cell cycle protein(s) involved in the G1/S transition which can be considered as the major control step of hepatocyte growth activity.
Moreover, a sequential proto-oncogene activation including c-fos/c-jun, c-myc/jun B/jun D/p53, and c-Ki-ras, has been established, corresponding to early entry in G1, progression in G1 and G1/S transition phases respectively. Further studies to elucidate their participation in the cell cycle-related protein complex formation and activation, will be very useful in better understanding general growth regulation.

References

Arion, D., Meijer, L., Brizuela, L. & Beach, D.(1988): Cdc2 is a component of the M phase-specific Histone H1 kinase: Evidence for identity with MPF. *Cell.* 55, 371-378.

Corral, M.,Tichoniky, L.,Guguen-Guillouzo, C.,Corcos D., Raymonjean, M., Paris, B., Kruh, J. & Defer, N. (1985): Expression of c-fos oncogene during hepatocarcinogenesis, liver regeneration and synchronized HTC cells. *Exp. Cell Res.* 160, 427-434.

Draetta, G., Piwnica-Worms, H., Morrison, D., Druker, B., Roberts, T. & Beach, D.(1988): Human cdc2 protein kinase is a major cell-cycle regulated tyrosine kinase substrate. *Nature*. 336, 738-744.

Elledge, S. J. & Spottswood, M. R.(1991): A new human p34 protein kinase, CDK2, identified by complementation of a cdc28 mutation in Saccharomyces cerevisiae, is a homolog of Xenopus Eg1. *EMBO J*. 10, 2653-2659.

Etienne, P. L., Baffet, G., Desvergne, B., Boisnard-Rissel, M., Glaise, D. & Guguen-Guillouzo, C.(1988): Transient expression of c-fos and constant expression of c-myc in freshly isolated and cultured normal adult rat hepatocytes. *Oncogene Res*, 3, 255-262.

Fang, F. & Newport, J. W.(1991): Evidence that the G1-S and G2-M transitions are controlled by different cdc2 proteins in higher eukaryotes. *Cell*. 66, 731-742.

Fabrikant, J. I.(1968): The kinetic of cellular proliferation in regenerating liver. *J. Cell. Biol.*36,551-565.

Friedman, D., Claus, T., Pilkis, S. & Pine, G.(1981): Hormonal regulation of DNA synthesis in primary cultures of adult rat hepatocytes- Action of glucagon. *Exp. Cell. Res*. 135, 283-290.

Grisham, J.W.(1962): A morphologic study of deoxyribonucleic acid synthesis and cell proliferation in regenerating rat liver; Autoradiography with Thymidine-H^3. *Cancer Res*. 22, 842-849.

Hasegawa, K., Watanabe, K. & Koga, M.(1982): Induction of mitosis in primary cultures of adult rat hepatocytes under serum free conditions. *Biochem. Biophys. Res. Commun.*104, 259-265.

Higgins, G. M. & Anderson, R. M.(1931): Exprimental pathology of liver; Restoration of the liver of the white rat following partial surgical removal. *Arch. Pathol.*12,186-202.

Ikeda, T., Sawada, N., Fujiniga, K., Minase, T. & Mori, M.(1989): C-H-ras gene is expressed at the G1 phase in primary cultures of hepatocytes. *Exp. Cell. Res.*185, 292-296.

Lee, M. G., Norbury, C. J., Spurr, N. K. & Nurse, P.(1988): Regulated expression and phosphorylation of a possible mammalian cell-cycle control protein. *Nature*. 333, 676-679.

McGowan, J. A.(1986): hepatocyte proliferation in culture: *Isolated and cultured Hepatocytes*. A. Guillouzo and C. Guguen-Guillouzo (eds.), p13-38. INSERM, Paris and John Libbey Eurotext, London.

Morello, D., Lavenu, A.& Babinet,.C. (1990): Differential regulation and expression of jun, c-fos and c-myc proto-oncogenes during mouse liver regeneration and after inhibition of protein synthesis. *Oncogene*. 5, 1511-1519.

Nurse, P. & Bissett, Y.(1982): Gene required in G1 for commitment to cell cycle and in G2 for control of mitosis in fission yeast. *Nature* 292, 558-560.

Paris, J., Le Guellec, R., Couturier, A., Le Guellec, K., Omilli, F., Camonis, J., MacNeill, S. & Philippe, M.(1991): Cloning by differential screening of a xenopus cDNA coding for a protein highly homologous to cdc2. *Proc. Natl. Acad. Sci. USA*. 88, 1039-1043.

Piggott, J., Rai, R. & Carter, B.(1982): A bifunctional gene product involved in two phases of the yeast cell cycle. *Nature*. 298, 391-393.

Richman, R. A., Claus, T. H., Pilkis, S. & Friedman, D. L.(1976): Hormonal stimulation of DNA synthesis in primary cultures of adult rat hepatocytes. *Proc. Natl. Acad. Sci. USA* 73, 3589-3593.

Sawada, N.(1989): Hepatocytes from old rats retain responsiveness of c-myc expression to EGF in primary culture but do not enter S phase. *Exp.Cell Res.* 5, 584-588.

Sobczak, J. & Duguet, M.(1986): Molecular biology of liver regeneration. *Biochimie* 68, 957-967.

Sobczack, J., Mechti, N., Tournier, M.F., Blanchard, J.M.,& Duguet, M.(1989): C-myc and c-fos gene regulation during mouse liver regeneration. *Oncogene.* 4, 1503-1508.

Thompson, N.L.,Mead, J.E., Braun, L., Goyette, M., Shank, P.R.& Fausto, N. (1986). Sequential proto-oncogene expression during rat liver regeneration. *Cancer Research.* 46, 3111-3117.

Thompson, C. B., Challoner, P. B., Neiman, P. E. & Groudine, M..(1985): Levels of c-myc oncogene mRNA are invariant throughout the cell cycle.*Nature.* 314, 363-366.

Oncogenes and liver regeneration

Joëlle Sobczak

Faculté Necker, INSERM U.75, service de Biochimie, 156 rue de Vaugirard, 75742 Paris Cedex 15, France

Since the early experiments by Goyette *et al* (1983), who showed that the c-*ras* proto-oncogene is activated during rat liver regeneration, a complex picture has emerged in which various oncogenes are sequentially expressed in the regenerating liver.
Cellular oncogenes were first identified as the normal cellular counterparts of retroviral transforming genes. In cancer cells, they are activated by a variety of mechanisms such as virus insertion, mutations and amplification (reviewed by Bishop, 1991). In normal cells, the protein products of cellular oncogenes are involved in the reception and transduction of mitogenic signals and in the regulation of cell proliferation (for comprehensive reviews, see Cantley *et al.*, 1991 ; Aaronson, 1991 and references therein). Accumulation of mRNAs and proteins encoded by cellular oncogenes was found to occur sequentially during the G0/G1/S transition of immortalized cell lines (*e.g.* rodent fibroblasts) and primary cultured cells (*e.g.* lymphocytes and hepatocytes).

Studying the expression of oncogenes during liver regeneration is of particular interest, since it is the simplest experimental model of normal dividing cells *in vivo*. Gene expression is usually studied during the first 30 hours after partial hepatectomy : cell division is observed exclusively among hepatocytes and not among other liver cell types, which divide at least 24 h later. It is therefore considered that mRNA and protein syntheses in the liver during this period concerns only hepatocytes. This should, however, be verified, whenever possible, by *in situ* techniques (*in situ* hybridization and immunohistochemistry) or by fractionation of hepatocytes and non-parenchymal cells prior to mRNA purification. The results are usually interpreted in terms of cell proliferation or DNA replication, but it should be checked that sham operation or experimental inflammation do not have the same effects.
We shall first describe those oncogenes activated during liver regeneration after partial hepatectomy in the rat or mouse, and then focus on the mechanisms of activation, taking the two proto-oncogenes c-*myc* and c-*fos* as examples. Finally, the biological significance of the results will be discussed.

Table 1 shows the sequential accumulation of proto-oncogene-encoded mRNAs during liver regeneration in the rat and mouse.

The genes first activated after partial hepatectomy correspond to the previously described early-response genes and belong to the *fos* and *jun* families ; they encode nuclear proteins engaged in a Fos-Jun heterodimer that is able to bind a specific DNA sequence, the AP1 site. In regenerating liver, the three genes c-*jun*, *jun* B and *jun* D are active and the mRNAs accumulate. c-*jun* and *jun*-B mRNAs are undetectable in normal liver but their levels rise rapidly after hepatectomy, as in cultured cells stimulated with growth factors (Ryseck *et al.*, 1988 ; Quantin *et al.*, 1988). *jun* D mRNA, however, is constitutively expressed in normal liver as well as in quiescent fibroblasts (Hirai *et al.*, 1989). Both results suggest that *jun* D plays a particular role in quiescent cells, although it may also be involved, like c-*jun* and *jun* B, in the transition toward the proliferative state.

Surprisingly, c-*jun* mRNA was detected in regenerating liver in both non-parenchymal cells and hepatocytes, by *in situ* hybridization and Northern blot analysis of purified cell populations (Alcorn *et al.* 1990). c-*jun* expression in hepatocytes occurs rapidly after partial hepatectomy and is followed, a few hours later, by DNA synthesis and cell division. The concomitant accumulation of c-*jun* and its expression in non-parenchymal cells is more difficult to interpret since these cells replicate two days later. It is not known whether c-*jun* exerts different functions in the two cell populations.

During liver regeneration, the c-*fos* mRNA level increases in parallel with that of c-*jun*, suggesting that the two genes are co-regulated. The other two *fos*-related genes *fos* B and *fra*-1 are not induced (Mohn *et al.*, 1990). Unfortunately, few if any data are available on Fos and Jun proteins in regenerating liver. Since c-*jun*, *jun* B and *jun* D are active, a combination of at least three heterodimers can be formed between each Jun protein and c-Fos, but which complex transactivates which target gene remains to be determined. Characterization of functional transcription activators should indeed provide valuable tools to study gene expression in regenerating liver. This point was recently illustrated by the identification of LRF-1, a nuclear protein able to form heterodimers with c-Jun and Jun B and to recognize cAMP responsive sequences (Hsu *et al.*, 1991). This finding showed that Jun proteins are not engaged in an obligatory complex with Fos, but can interact with other proteins and form new transactivators.

Some targets of the Fos-Jun transactivators have been identified. They include a replication-dependent histone gene and the metalloprotease transin gene, which may reflect a role for the activation of *fos*, *jun* and related genes in G1/S transition and extracellular matrix remodeling, respectively. *Fos* and *jun* activation may also trigger a cascade of transcriptional activation which starts with the activation of c-*myc*.

Early c-*myc* mRNA accumulation is observed in regenerating liver, as well as after sham operation and during the acute-phase response, although to a lesser extent (see Table 1). This suggests that c-*myc* plays a role in both the acute-phase response and liver cell proliferation. However, we do not know yet whether c-*myc* mRNA and protein are present in the same cell type during regeneration or during the acute-phase response.

The mechanisms governing c-*myc* mRNA accumulation have been investigated. Transcriptional activation and mRNA stabilization are responsible for c-*myc* mRNA accumulation during liver regeneration (Sobczak *et al.*, 1989a ; Morello *et al.*, 1990), but the half-life of this mRNA is unknown, given the difficulty of measuring this parameter *in vivo*. Conversely, only mRNA stabilization appears to occur during the acute-phase response (Sobczak *et al.*, 1989 a).

c-Myc is a nuclear phospho-protein which can interact with Max and/or p105^{RB} in a transcriptional activator complex. Its role in DNA replication was hypothesized some years ago but remains controversial. It is, however, supported by the second peak of c-*myc* mRNA accumulation 18-20h after hepatectomy (see Table 1), although we do not know whether this occurs in replicating hepatocytes. *In situ* hybridization failed to reveal preferential localisation of the c-*myc* mRNA at any time after hepatectomy, and immunohistochemistry using c-Myc-specific antibodies was no more successful (MF Tournier and J. Sobczak, unpublished results). The function of c-Myc protein during liver regeneration remains to be established.

The gene encoding p53 is activated next, at a time corresponding to late G_1 in proliferating hepatocytes. p53 is a nuclear phosphoprotein acting as an anti-oncogene and as a transcriptional activator (rewieved by Weinberg, 1991 ; Marshall, 1991). It is transiently accumulated at 12-15h post-hepatectomy (Thompson *et al.*, 1986), suggesting a role in the modulation of hepatocyte proliferation *in vivo*.

Finally, several mRNAs accumulate during S-phase including c-Ha-*ras* and c-Ki-*ras* (see Table 1). c-Ha-*ras* mRNA is accumulated in hepatocytes but not in non-parenchymal cells (Silverman *et al.*, 1989). This further confirms that c-Ha-*ras* mRNA accumulation is in some way related to hepatocyte proliferation. $p21^{ras}$ is a G-protein anchored on the plasma membrane (reviewed by Downward, 1990). Since it dissociates from the membrane of isolated hepatocytes upon stimulation with alpha1-adrenergic agonists, it was suggested that $p21^{ras}$ is involved in the transduction of mitogenic signals mediated by alpha1-receptors (Cruise *et al.*, 1989). Data concerning the synthesis of $p21^{ras}$ in hepatocytes during liver regeneration should give new insight into the functions of this protein during DNA replication.
raf 1 and *ets* 2 mRNAs are accumulated in parallel with c-Ha-*ras* mRNA in regenerating liver. A- and c-*raf* 1 oncogenes encode cytoplasmic Ser-Thr protein kinases, which are activated by mitogenic stimuli via G protein-coupled receptors and/or via Tyr-kinase-associated receptors (reviewed in Bishop, 1991). Unfortunately, neither Raf kinase activity nor its translocation to the nucleus have yet been investigated in regenerating liver. Data concerning the *ets*-2 - encoded protein are also sparse and the function of this transcriptional activator in regenerating liver is still unknown.

In summary, numerous oncogenes are activated during the liver regeneration process ; they obviously play a role in the regulation of hepatocyte and non-parenchymal cell proliferation, but several points remain obscure. The first relates to the mechanism of oncogene activation. In the case of c-*myc* and c-*fos*, a complex mechanism of transcriptional regulation has emerged. Both genes are actively transcribed in regenerating liver as a result of frequent initiation and efficient elongation. In normal liver, however, the initiation of transcription is reduced compared to regenerating liver and elongation is completely blocked, which results in the absence of detectable mRNAs (Sobczak *et al.* 1989, Morello *et al.* 1990). Regulation of transcription elongation could be a common mechanism for transiently induced oncogenes. The second point concerns the proteins encoded by oncogenes, whose functions and properties in normal cells *in vivo* are still poorly documented. The identification of LRF1 (Hsu *et al.*, 1991) and the characterisation of a new transcriptional complex on the c-*fos* promoter (De Belle *et al.*, 1991) confirms that regenerating liver is a good experimental model for the study of oncogene regulation. Ongoing work will no doubt provide new insights into the molecular regulation of hepatocyte proliferation *in vivo*.

Table 1

oncogene	animal	mRNA level		transcription rate	references
		fold induction (time#)	period of time*	fold induction (time#)	
c-jun	mouse	13/S.O. (2h)	0,5 - 2h	2 (2h)	Alcorn et al., 1990
	mouse	20/S.O.; 50/N.L. (1h)	0,5 - 4h	6 (0,5h)	Morello et al., 1990
	rat	20/S.O. (0,5h)	0,5 - 8h	ND	Mohn et al., 1990
jun B	mouse	1,5/S.O. (2h)	0,5 - 2h	ND	Alcorn et al., 1990
	mouse	20/S.O.; 50/N.L. (1h)	0,5 - 4h	3 (0,5h)	Morello et al., 1990
	rat	20/N.L. (0,5h)	0,5 - 8h	ND	Mohn et al., 1990
jun D	mouse	10/N.L. (1h)	0,5 - 4h	ND	Morello et al., 1990
	rat	2/N.L. (1h)	0 - 24 h	ND	Mohn et al., 1990
c-fos	mouse	2,5/S.O.; 12/N.L. (0,5h)	0,2 - 8h	ND	Kruijer et al., 1986
	mouse	50/S.O.; 50/N.L. (6h)	2 - 6h	8 (2h)	Sobczak et al., 1989a
	rat	4/S.O. (0,25h)	0,25 - 4h	ND	Thompson et al., 1986
	rat	2/S.O. (8h)	8h	ND	Thompson et al., 1986
c-myc	rat	10-15/N.L. (1h)	1 - 8h	ND	Makino et al., 1984
	rat	5/N.L. (18h)	12 - 24h	ND	Goyette et al., 1984
	rat	5/S.O. (2h)	0,5 - 4h	ND	Thompson et al., 1986
	rat	5/S.O. (8h)	8h	ND	Thompson et al., 1986
	rat	2/S.O.; 10/N.L. (1h)	0,5 - 8h	ND	Sobczak et al., 1989b
	rat	10/S.O.; 20/N.L. (20h)	20h	ND	Sobczak et al., 1989b
	mouse	50/N.L. (6h)	2 - 40h	6 (2h)	Sobczak et al., 1989a
	mouse	2/S.O.; 10/N.L. (2h)	1 - 2h	3-5 (0,5h)	Morello et al., 1990
p53	rat	5/S.O. (8-12h)	4 - 24h	ND	Thompson et al., 1986
c-Ha-ras	rat	3/N.L. (18-24h)	12 - 72h	ND	Goyette et al., 1983
c-Ki-ras	rat	10/S.O.; 20-50/N.L. (24h)	12 - 96h	ND	Goyette et al., 1984
A-raf-1	rat	3-5/N.L. (24h)	3 - 72h	ND	Silverman et al., 1989
c-raf-1	rat	3-5/N.L. (24h)	3 - 72h	ND	Silverman et al., 1989
ets-2	mouse	10/S.O. (4h)	2 - 24h	ND	Bhat et al., 1987

\# time after hepatectomy (hours)
* period after hepatectomy during which the mRNA is detectable
S.O. : versus sham-operated controls
N.L. : versus normal liver
ND : not determined

References

Aaronson, S.T. (1991): Growth factor and cancer. *Science* 254, 1146-1152.

Alcorn, J.A., Feitelberg, S.P. & Brenner, D.A. (1990): Transient induction of c-*jun* during hepatic regeneration. *Hepatology* 11,909-915.

De Belle, I., Walker, P.R., Smith, I.C.P. & Sikorska, M. (1991): Identification of a multiprotein complex interacting with the c-*fos* serum response element. *Mol. Cell. Biol.* 11,2752-2759.

Bhat, N.K., Fisher, R.J., Fujiwara, S., Ascione, R. & Papas T.S. (1987): Temporal and tissue specific expression of mouse *ets* genes. *Proc. Natl. Acad. Sci. USA* 84, 3161-3165.

Bishop, J.M. (1991): Molecular themes in oncogenesis. *Cell* 64, 235-248.

Cantley, L.C., Auger, K.A., Carpenter, C., Duckworth, B., Graziani, A., Kapeller, R. & Soltoff, S. (1991): Oncogenes and signal transduction. *Cell* 64, 281-302.

Cruise, J.L., Muga, S.J., Lee, Y. & Michalopoulos, G.K. (1989): Regulation of hepatocyte growth : Alpha-1 adrenergic receptor and *ras* p21 changes in liver regeneration. *J. Cell. Physiol.* 140, 195-201.

Downward, J. (1990): The *ras* superfamily of small GTP-binding proteins. *TIBS* 15, 469-477.

Goyette, M., Petropoulos, C.J., Shank, P.R. & Fausto, N. (1983): Expression of a cellular oncogene during liver regeneration. *Science* 219, 510-512.

Goyette, M., Petropoulos, C.J., Shank, P.R. & Fausto, N. (1984): Regulated transcription of c-Ki-*ras* and c-*myc* during compensatory growth of rat liver. *Mol. Cell. Biol.* 4, 1493-1498.

Hirai, S.I., Ryseck, R.P., Mechta, F., Bravo, R. & Yaniv, M. (1989): Characterisation of *jun* D : a new member of the *jun* proto-oncogene family. *EMBO J.* 8, 1433-1439.

Hsu, J.C., Laz, T., Mohn, K.L. & Taub, R. (1991): Identification of LRF-1, a leucine zipper protein that is rapidly and highly induced in regenerating rat liver. *Proc. Natl. Acad. Sci. USA* 88, 3511-3515.

Kruijer, W., Skelly, H., Botteri, F., van der Putten, H., Barber, J.R., Verma, I.M. & Leffert, H.L. (1986): Proto-oncogene expression in regenerating liver is stimulated in cultures of primary adult rat hepatocytes.*J. Biol. Chem.* 261, 7929-7933.

Marshall, C.J. (1991): Tumor suppressor genes. *Cell* 64, 313-326.

Makino, R., Hayashi, K. & Sugimura, T. (1984): c-*myc* transcript is induced in rat liver at a very early stage of regeneration or by cycloheximide treatment. *Nature* 310, 697-698.

Mohn, K.L., Laz, T.M., Melby, A.E. & Taub, R. (1990): Immediate-early gene expression differs between regenerating liver, insulin-stimulated H-35 cells and mitogen-stimulated Balb/c 3T3 cells. *J. Biol. Chem.* 265, 21914-21921.

Morello, D., Lavenu, A. & Babinet, C. (1990): Differential regulation and expression of *jun*, c-*fos* and c-*myc* proto-oncogenes during mouse liver regeneration and after inhibition of protein synthesis. *Oncogene* 5, 1511-1519.

Quantin, B. & Breathnach, R. (1988): Epidermal growth factor stimulates the transcription of the c-*jun* proto-oncogene in rat fibroblasts. *Nature* 334, 538-539.

Ryseck, R.P., Hirai, S.I., Yaniv, M. & Bravo, R. (1988): Transcriptional activation of c-*jun* during the G0/G1 transition in mouse fibroblasts. *Nature* 334, 535-537.

Silverman, J.A., Zurlo, J., Watson, M.A. & Yager, J.D. (1989): Expression of c-*raf*-1 and A-*raf*-1 during regeneration of rat liver following surgical partial hepatectomy. *Mol. Carcinogenesis* 2, 63-67.

Sobczak, J., Mechti, N., Tournier, M.F., Blanchard, J.M. & Duguet, M. (1989a): c-*myc* and c-*fos* gene regulation during mouse liver regeneration. *Oncogene* 4, 1503-1508.

Sobczak, J., Tournier, M.F., Lotti, A.M. & Duguet, M. (1989b): Gene expression in regenerating liver in relation to cell proliferation and stress. *Eur. J. Biochem.* 180, 49-53.

Thompson, N.L., Mead, J.E., Braun, L., Goyette, M., Shank, P.R. & Fausto, N. (1986): Sequential proto-oncogene expression during rat liver regeneration. *Cancer Res.* 46, 3111-3117.

Weinberg, R.A. (1991): Tumor suppressor genes. Science 254, 1138-1146.

Liver Regeneration. Eds D. Bernuau, G. Feldmann. John Libbey Eurotext, Paris © 1992, pp. 77-84.

Regulation of liver growth by transforming growth factor alpha

Nelson Fausto

Department of Pathology and Laboratory Medicine, Brown University, Providence, Rhode Island 02912, USA

The transforming growth factors alpha (TGFα) and beta (TGFβ) were originally described as peptides which could act synergistically to transform non-neoplastic rat kidney fibroblasts (NRK) in culture and make them grow in soft agar (Anzano et al., 1983). Further studies showed that these peptides had completely different structures and had similar, different or opposite effects on cell growth and transformation depending on cell type (Marquardt et al., 1984; Roberts et al., 1985). The name "transforming" is also not appropriate as TGFα and β are produced by normal cells, both embryonic and adult, and participate in a multiplicity of physiological activities (Derynck, 1988; Roberts and Sporn, 1986).

TGFα is produced by proliferating normal cells and by many transformed cells and tumors. For epithelial tumors, overexpression of TGFα may be a necessary but not sufficient step in the transformation process (Derynck, 1988). In contrast, epithelial cells generally lose sensitivity to the inhibitory effects of TGFβ at what appears to be an early stage of transformation (Moses et al., 1990). These altered cells became capable of growing in an environment that prevents proliferation of normal cells.

TGFα is a mitogen for epithelial cells including hepatocytes, while TGFβ1 generally functions as an inhibitor of DNA synthesis (Mead and Fausto, 1989; Fausto, 1991). In the regenerating liver TGFα and β have opposite effects as respectively an autocrine stimulator and a paracrine inhibitor of hepatocyte proliferation (Braun et al., 1988). During hepatocarcinogenesis, TGFβ may function as a selective agent that permits the growth of cells which overexpress TGFα but inhibits the replication of normal hepatocytes (Braun et al., 1990; Nakatsukasa et al., 1991).

<u>General properties of TGFα</u>

TGFα is synthesized from a precursor of 160 amino acids and is cleaved to a 50-amino acid peptide (human) that contains 3 disulphide bonds (Roberts and Sporn, 1985). The sequence and structure of the peptide is remarkably conserved between rodents and humans, especially in the cysteine-rich carboxy end of the precursor. TGFα shares 35% homology with EGF and binds to and phosphorylates the EGF receptor although the binding properties of the 2 ligands may differ. These 2 factors are the prototypes of a family which includes the vaccinia, pox virus and Shope fibroma factors, amphiregulin, the CRIPTO and NOTCH genes and heparin binding-EGF, among others. These peptides have the 3 disulphide bonds present in EGF and TGFα and share a stretch of 10 amino acids in one of the disulphide loops.

TGFα and its receptor during liver development

Expression of TGFα in rat liver is developmentally regulated. The peptide is detectable in rat liver at 20 days of gestation and decreases to low adult levels by about the second week after birth. The hepatic concentrations are approximately 24-70 pg/mg of protein from the last 2 days of gestation until 14 days post birth, and decrease to approximately 3 pg/mg of protein thereafter (Brown et al., 1990). Expression of the mRNA in the liver is highest during the first post-natal week and decreases to very low levels thereafter (Fausto et al., 1990; Evarts et al., 1992). During the last 3 days of gestation in the rat, the number of EGF/TGFα receptors in the liver increases sharply, and reaches the high adult levels by the twenty-first day (last day of gestation). In fetal and hepatocytes, (as well as in adults) EGF and TGFα compete for the same receptor site, although the affinity for TGFα is generally lower (Gruppuso, 1989). As EGF is not made in fetal and adult rat liver and prepro-EGF mRNA is detectable in other tissues (Rall et al., 1985) only after birth (at 2 weeks in kidneys and 3-4 weeks in salivary glands), it is most likely that TGFα is the physiological ligand for the EGF/TGFα receptor during rat liver development.

TGFα as an hepatocyte mitogen: liver regeneration and cell culture studies

TGFα synthesis increases in rat liver hepatocytes during liver regeneration. TGFα mRNA changes are first detectable 4-8 h after partial hepatectomy and reach a maximum of about 8-10 fold above normal levels (sham-operated animals) at 20-24 h (Mead and Fausto, 1989). These changes slightly precede the major wave of DNA synthesis in the regenerating liver. The amounts of TGFα in the regenerating rat liver (measured by RIA with an antibody that recognizes the mature form of the peptide) approximately double between 12 and 18 h after partial hepatectomy (FitzGerald et al., submitted).

TGFα is a potent stimulator of DNA synthesis for rat and human hepatocytes in primary culture and is generally 25-200 percent more active than EGF in its stimulatory effect (Mead and Fausto, 1989; Ismail et al., 1991). In cultured hepatocytes the addition of TGFα causes the initiation of a proliferative program (Brenner et al., 1989) and a wave of DNA synthesis with a maximum at 48-72 h (Mead and Fausto, 1989). In the replicating cells (both in rat and mouse hepatocytes), there is an increase of TGFα mRNA and release of the peptide in the culture medium. Neither the mRNA nor peptide levels change in nonstimulated cultures, where they are barely detectable (Mead and Fausto, 1989). Thus both in vivo and in culture, TGFα mRNA and the peptide increase in hepatocytes which have entered the cell cycle and progress to DNA replication.

Does EGF participate in liver regeneration in vivo?

EGF is a potent stimulator of DNA synthesis for hepatocytes in in vitro systems, and is routinely used as a growth factor in primary cultures of hepatocytes. However, it has been difficult to establish a physiological role for EGF in the regulation of rat liver regeneration in vivo because the factor and its RNA are not synthesized by normal or regenerating livers. Furthermore, EGF is not detectable by RIA in the portal blood of normal or partially hepatectomized rats (Olsen et al., 1988). Sialoadenectomy has no effect on rat liver regeneration while duodenectomy (salivary glands and Brunner glands in the duodenum are sites where EGF is produced in rodents) has a very slight effect on DNA synthesis after partial hepatectomy. Nevertheless, administration of EGF together with insulin or glucagon increases liver DNA synthesis in normal or partially hepatectomized rats (Bucher et al., 1978; Webber and Fausto, in preparation). These data indicate that EGF may not be a major participant of rat liver regeneration in vivo but it has a strong effect on hepatocyte replication when injected into the animal or added to cells in culture. However, it is possible that in mice, EGF may play a significant role in regulating liver regeneration in vivo. In these animals, sialoadenectomy causes a decrease in plasma EGF and leads to a considerable delay in the peak of DNA synthesis after partial hepatectomy (Noguchi et al., 1991). This delay can be eliminated by supplementation of EGF to sialoadenectomized rats. These experiments suggest that in mice EGF could function as an endocrine regulator of liver regeneration (Naguchi et al., 1991).

EGF/TGFα receptor (EGFR) changes during liver regeneration

Earp and O'Keefe (1981) have shown that the number of EGFR decreases during rat liver regeneration, an observation confirmed in many other laboratories (Gruppuso et al., 1990). Only the number but not the affinity of EGFR changes after partial hepatectomy. TGFα and EGF compete for the same M_r=170,000 protein and, although TGFα is a more potent stimulator of DNA replication, it binds with lower affinity than EGF (Gruppuso et al., 1990). Because the magnitude of EGF and TGFα effects on hepatocyte proliferation do not directly correlate with the binding affinity of the ligands, it is possible that EGF and TGFα receptor complexes are processed in different ways or with different efficiency by the hepatocyte (Ebner and Derynck, 1991). In A431 cells, studies with a monoclonal antibody (13A9) raised against the receptor suggest that each ligand may induce different receptor conformations which may result in differing biological effects (Winkler et al., 1989). Another possibility is that the receptor may contain distinct binding sites, one for each ligand. Conformational changes in the receptor after binding by one ligand may cause competition or displacement of the other ligand. However, it is not known whether similar findings would be obtained with hepatocytes or other cell types.

The decrease in EGFR number during rat liver regeneration is not in dispute, but various hypotheses that attempt to explain the mechanisms responsible for the change have been offered. After partial hepatectomy or following the intraportal injection of EGF, the amount of EGFR mRNA increases during the first 2-4 h (Johansson and Andersson, 1990). In this situation, it is likely that changes in receptor number are a consequence of increased turnover. The data on EGFR mRNA levels at later stages of liver regeneration are conflicting, with reports concluding that they decrease (Johansson et al., 1990; Bartles et al., 1991) or increase (Mead and Fausto, 1989; Johnson et al., 1988) at 18-24 h after partial hepatectomy. Depending on the direction of the change observed in EGFR mRNA, the decrease in receptor number is explained as resulting from either lack of synthesis of receptor protein (decrease in EGFR mRNA) or, in an opposite way, as ligand induced down-regulation and turnover (increase in EGFR mRNA). Johansson et al. (1990) made the interesting observation that in regenerating rat liver, the number of EGF binding sites in prelysosomal endosomes is much less reduced than the membrane receptor sites. This suggests that endogenously produced TGFα could be bound to the receptor in intracellular compartments. However, it is not known what proportion of TGFα synthesized in the regenerating rat liver remains in intracellular compartments, is anchored to the hepatocyte plasma membrane or is cleaved into the 50 amino acid peptide (or partially cleaved to other forms) and released. Receptor dynamics and the relationship between the levels of receptor protein and its mRNA would differ significantly if TGFα effects were exerted by membrane anchored forms instead of the free, mature peptide (Brachman et al., 1989).

In mice, there is an increase in EGFR binding after partial hepatectomy with a peak at 8 h (Noguchi et al., 1992). As DNA synthesis increases (between 24 and 48 h), the levels of EGFR binding sharply decrease. The amounts of EGFR RNA are approximately 3 fold higher than normal at 8 h after partial hepatectomy, an increase due primarily to enhanced transcription (Naguchi et al., 1992). These data are consistent with the notion that EGFR is initially increased and then down regulated during the regenerative process as a consequence of changes in ligand concentration. As discussed above, circulating EGF in addition to TGFα synthesized in the liver may be important physiological ligands for the receptor in mice.

Regulation of liver growth and tumorigenesis in TGFα transgenic mice

The expression of TGFα in the regenerating liver is a transient event that is associated with the major wave of DNA synthesis. It becomes important to determine what effects the constitutive overexpression of the gene *vivo* might have on liver growth. Transgenic mice carrying TGFα constructs are ideally suited for these studies and lines that overexpress human TGFα have been established. Transgenic mouse lines in which the human TGFα gene is controlled by the mouse metallothionein I promoter proved to be particularly useful for analysis of the role of TGFα in normal and neoplastic liver growth.

Both Sandgren et al. (1990) and Jhappan et al (1990) found that TGFα overexpression causes an increase in liver mass in young animals (2-6 weeks old). The liver weight/body weight ratio and the amount of DNA/mg of protein in the liver of the transgenic animals was 25-90% higher than in non-transgenic controls of the same age (Sandgren et al., 1990; Fausto, in preparation). In older animals the difference in liver weights between transgenic and non-transgenic mice was much smaller, suggesting that the TGFα effect is most important during the postnatal growth period. The major difference in the findings reported by these two groups of investigators is that the incidence of tumor in the CD1 transgenic mice used by Jhappan et al. (1990) was very high (about 80%) while it was low in the strain (C57Bl/6 x 5JL, F2) used by Sandgren et al. (1990). In the CD1 transgenic mice tumors appeared after 12 months of age, but studies with older animals of the 57BL/6 x 5JL strain have not yet been reported. The difference in tumor incidence between these strains may simply reflect the age at which the animals were examined. However it is of interest that normal CD1 mice have a 5-8% spontaneous incidence of hepatocellular tumors (all benign tumors appearing after one year) while the incidence of spontaneous tumors is negligible in the strain used by Sandgren et al. (1990). In CD1 transgenic mice, about 30% of the tumors were hepatocellular carcinomas and the rest were adenomas. All carcinomas overexpressed TGFα and were negative for γGT or G6Pase activity. Most of the carcinomas but no adenomas were AFP positive (Lee et al., submitted).

The increase in liver weight in the young transgenic animals is caused by liver cell hypertrophy, changes in ploidy, and hyperplasia. The livers of these animals have very high mitotic activity (as indicated by labeling index data obtained after 3H-thymidine infusion for 3 and 7 days) and higher DNA content/mg tissue than nontransgenic mice (Fausto, in preparation). The most obvious morphologic change in the liver of the transgenic animals is centrolobular hypertrophy,similar to that observed after phenobarbital administration. Immunohistochemical staining with an antibody that detects the TGFα precursor molecule showed by that cells overexpressing TGFα in the liver of transgenic mice have a patchy distribution with heavily stained hepatocytes forming nests located in centrolobular or periportal areas (Lee et al., submitted). Northern blot analysis, immunohistochemistry and *in situ* hybridization techniques demonstrated that the tumors formed in these animals generally had a much higher level of TGFα expression than the surrounding tissue (Lee et al., submitted; Takagi et al., submitted). On the other hand, there were areas of very high TGFα expression by apparently normal hepatocytes suggesting that increased expression of TGFα by itself may not be sufficient for transformation (Lee et al., submitted).

Could the development of liver tumors in TGFα transgenic mice be the result of transgene overexpression alone? This is an unlikely possibility because the tumors formed in these animals are focal, take at least 12 months to develop and generally have higher levels of TGFα expression than the surrounding tissue. More likely liver neoplasia in TGFα transgenic mice requires the interaction between TGFα overexpression and some other events. It is then plausible to suggest that the transgene functions as a promoter rather than an initiator of carcinogenesis by inducing the proliferation of already altered cells, by increasing the risk for the development of genetic alterations in normal cells or by interacting with other growth factors overexpressed by transformed cells. TGFα mRNA expression was increased in 17/25 (68%) tumors while IGFII and c-myc mRNA were enhanced in 75% and 37% of the tumors (Takagi et al., submitted). So far, neither *ras* nor p53 mutations or deletions have been found to occur at a higher frequency in the tumors. A potentially interesting clue to the pathogenesis of the tumors is that they develop in high frequency in CD1 males but rarely in females. This difference is not due to the number of liver EGFR sites in transgenic mice of different sexes but is probably related to hormonal changes. The incidence of liver tumors was reduced about 7 fold in castrated transgenic animals and was increased by about 6 fold by ovariectomy (Takagi et al., submitted).

Establishment of cultures of hepatocytes from TGFα transgenic mice

Hepatocytes from TGFα transgenic mice can be maintained in primary culture in serum free media without any growth factors and undergo at least 1-3 rounds of synchronous replication (Wu et al., submitted). These cells secrete active TGFα in the culture medium and show an increase in the mRNA for the endogenous murine TGFα as they replicate. Addition of either EGF or HGF to the medium does not enhance the level of DNA synthesis. Thus, hepatocytes from TGFα transgenic animals have the capacity to replicate autonomously in culture (within certain limits) most likely because of TGFα autocrine activity. By maintaining the cells in serum-free medium without growth factors but in the presence of nicotinamide, several cell lines have been developed with hepatocytes from TGFα transgenic animals. Preliminary results indicate that some of these lines retain differentiated hepatocyte traits and morphology for at least 2-3 months, do not grow in soft agar and are not tumorigenic in nude mice (Wu, et al., submitted).

TGFα expression during hepatocarcinogenesis and in liver tumors in non-transgenic animals and humans

Urinary TGFα excretion has been reported by Yeh et al. (1987) to be much higher in patients with hepatocellular carcinoma than in normal controls, although there is large individual variation. They found a significant difference in TGF α excretion (expressed as $\mu g TGF\alpha/g$ creatinine) between patients with primary liver cancer and controls. The same authors reported that urinary EGF levels were not changed in these patients and showed that EGF/TGFα ratios in the urine of patients with hepatocellular carcinomas were significantly decreased. On the basis of these results they suggested that the measurement of urinary TGFα may be a useful tumor marker, particularly for patients with hepatocellular carcinomas who have low serum alphafetoprotein levels (Yeh et al., 1987).

Studies with liver epithelial cells which can function as precursors to hepatocellular carcinomas indicate that transformation of these cells is generally associated with increased TGFα gene expression (Grisham et al, 1990). As shown in various laboratories, immortalized nontumorigenic liver epithelial cells do not generally produce TGFα. However, their transformation by chemicals, oncogene transfection or manipulation of culture conditions causes an increase in TGFα mRNA and the secretion of active peptide in the culture medium (Laird and Fausto, in preparation). In the WB liver epithelial cell line extensively analyzed by Grisham, Tsao and their colleagues, TGFα expression and tumorigenicity cosegregate in many different clonal lines (Lee et al., 1991). The correlation between overexpression of TGFα and tumorigenic capacity is particularly strong in clones that overexpress c-*myc* in addition to TGFα. Although the expression of c-*myc* and TGFα are likely to be independently controlled, they act synergistically in promoting tumorigenesis. One possibility is that high levels of MYC sensitize the cells to the mitogenic effect of TGFα. These studies are further confirmation that TGFα functions through an autocrine loop to regulate liver growth. TGFα overexpression appears to be an important but not sufficient even in the development of liver tumors in rodents. Some preliminary data suggest that this may also be the case in humans (Collier et al., 1991; Hsia et al., 1991).

Conclusions: Role of TGFα in liver regeneration and hepatocarcinogenesis

1. TGFα expression appears to be required for the progression of hepatocytes from G1 to S. Transient expression of TGFα occurs in the regenerating liver after partial hepatectomy and in hepatocytes in primary culture which have been stimulated to undergo DNA synthesis.
2. Maximal TGFα expression in the liver after partial hepatectomy, CCl_4 or galactosamine injury occurs in conjunction with or shortly preceding DNA synthesis by only a few hours. In contrast, the peak of HGF expression occurs within 12 h of injury after CCl_4 or galactosamine administration, preceding the wave of hepatocyte DNA synthesis by 1-4 days.
3. It is possible that HGF is an early signal for liver mitogenesis (especially after liver injury) while TGFα is required for hepatocyte replication and cell cycle completion.
4. Overexpression of TGFα in transgenic mice causes increased liver mass and greatly enhances hepatocyte proliferation in younger animals. Approximately 80% of TGFα transgenic mice develop liver tumors at 13-15 months of age.
5. TGFα overexpression is probably required but not in itself sufficient for the development of liver tumors in TGFα transgenic mice and non-transgenic rodents.
6. Preliminary data suggest that TGFα may be involved in the formation of human hepatocellular carcinomas.

REFERENCES

Anzano, M.A., Roberts, A.B., Smith, J.M., Sporn, M.B. and DeLarco, J.E. (1983): Sarcoma growth factor from conditioned medium is composed of both type alpha and type beta transforming growth factors. *Proc. Natl. Acad. Sci. U.S.A.* 80, 6264-6268.
Bartles, J.R., Zhang, L.Q., Verheyen, E.M., Hospodar, K.S., Nehme, C.L. and Fayos, B.E. (1991): Decreases in the relative concentrations of specific hepatocyte plasma membrane proteins during liver regeneration: down-regulation or dilution? *Dev. Biol.* 143, 258-270.
Brachman, R., Lindquist, P.B., Nagashima, M., Kohr, W., Lipari, T., Napier, M. and Derynck, R. (1989): Transmembrane TGF-α precursors activate EGF/TGFα receptors. *Cell* 56, 691-700.
Braun, L., Mead, J.E., Panzica, M., Mikumo, R., Bell, G.I. and Fausto, N. (1988): Elevation of transforming growth factor-beta mRNA during liver regeneration: A possible paracrine mechanism of growth regulation. *Proc. Natl. Acad. Sci. U.S.A.* 85, 1534-1538.
Braun, L., Gruppuso, P., Mikumo, R. and Fausto, N. (1990): TGF-β in liver carcinogenesis: mRNA expression and growth effects. *Cell Growth Differ.* 1, 103-111.
Brenner, D.A., Koch, K.S. and Leffert, H.L. (1989): Transforming growth factor-α stimulates proto-oncogene c-*jun* expression and a mitogenic program in primary

cultures of adult rat hepatocytes. *DNA* 8, 279-285.
Brown, P.I., Lam, R., Lakshmanan, J. and Fisher, D.A. (1990): Transforming growth factor alpha in developing rats. *Am. J. Physiol.* 259, E256-E260.
Bucher, N.L.R., Patel, U. and Cohen, S. (1978): Hormonal factors concerned with liver regeneration. In *Hepatotrophic factors, Ciba Foundation Symposium No. 55* (New Series), pp. 95-107. Amsterdam: Elsevier.
Collier, J.D., Guo, K., Gullick, W.J., Challen, C., Burt, A.D. and Basendine, M.F. (1991): Transforming growth factor alpha (TGF-α): a role in human hepatocarcinogenesis by an autocrine mechanism? *Hepatology* 14, 110A.
Derynck, R. (1988): Transforming growth factor α. *Cell* 54, 593-595.
Earp, H.S. and O'Keefe, E.J. (1981): Epidermal growth factor receptor number decreases during rat liver regeneration. *J. Clin. Invest.* 67, 1580-1583.
Ebner, R. and Derynck, R. (1991): Epidermal growth factor and transforming growth factor-α: differential intracellular routing and processing of ligand-receptor complexes. *Cell Regulation* 2, 599-612.
Evarts, R.P., Nakatsukasa, H., Marsden, E.R., Hu, Z. and Thorgeirsson, S. (1992): Expression of transforming growth factor-alpha in regenerating liver and during hepatic differentiation. *Mol. Carcinogenesis* 5, 25-31.
Fausto, N., Mead, J.E., Gruppuso, P.A. and Braun, L. (1990): TGFβ in liver development, regeneration and carcinogenesis. *Ann. N.Y. Acad. Sci.* 592, 231-242.
Fausto, N. (1991): Growth factors in liver development, regeneration and carcinogenesis. *Prog. Growth Factor Res.* 3, 219-234.
Grisham, J.W., Tsao, M-S., Lee, D.C. and Earp, H.S. (1990): Sequential changes in epidermal growth factor receptor/ligand function in cultured rat liver epithelial cells transformed chemically *in vitro*. *Pathobiology* 58, 3-14.
Gruppuso, P.A. (1989): Expression of hepatic transforming growth factor receptors during late gestation in the fetal rat. *Endocrinology* 125, 3037-3043.
Gruppuso, P.A., Mead, J.E. and Fausto N. (1990): Transforming growth factor receptors in liver regeneration following partial hepatectomy in the rat. *Cancer Res.* 50, 1464-1469.
Hsia, C.D., Axiotis, C.A., DiBisceglie, A.M. and Tabor, E. (1991): Co-expression of transforming growth factor-α and hepatitis B surface antigen in the same hepatocytes of human liver tissue adjacent to hepatocellular carcinoma. *Hepatology* 14, 109A.
Ismail, T., Howl, J., Wheatley, M., McMaster, P., Neuberger, J.M. and Strain, A.J. (1991): Growth of normal human hepatocytes in primary culture: Effect of hormones and growth factors on DNA synthesis. *Hepatology* 14, 1076-1082.
Jhappan, C., Stahle, C., Harkins, R.N., Fausto, N., Smith, G.H. and Merlino, G.T. (1990): TGFα overexpression in transgenic mice induces liver neoplasia and abnormal development of the mammary gland and pancreas. *Cell* 61, 1137-1146.
Johansson, S. and Andersson, G.(1990): Similar induction of the hepatic EGF receptor in vivo by EGF and partial hepatectomy. *Biochem. Biophys. Res. Commun.* 166, 661-666.
Johansson, S., Andersson, N. and Andersson, G. (1990): Pretranslational and postranslational regulation of the EGF receptor during the prereplicative phase of liver regeneration. *Hepatology* 12, 533-541.
Johnson, A.C., Garfield, S.F., Merlino, G.T. and Pastan, I. (1988): Expression of epidermal growth factor receptor proto-oncogene mRNA in regenerating rat liver. *Biochem. Biophys. Res. Commun.* 150, 412-418.
Lee, L.W., Raymond, V.W., Tsao, M-S., Lee, D.C., Earp, H.S. and Grisham, J.W. (1991): Clonal cosegregation of tumorigenicity with overexpression of c-*myc* and transforming growth factor α genes in chemically transformed rat liver epithelial cells. *Cancer Res.* 51, 5238-5244.
Marquardt, H., Hunkapiller, M.W., Hood, L. and Todaro, G.J. (1984): Rat transforming growth factor type 1: Structure and relation to epidermal growth factor. *Science* 223, 1079-1082.
Mead, J.E. and Fausto, N. (1989): Transforming growth factor α may be a physiological regulator of liver regeneration by means of an autocrine mechanism.

Proc. Natl. Acad. Sci. U.S.A. 86, 1558-1562.

Moses, H.L., Yang, E. Y. and Pietenpol, J.E. (1990): TGFβ stimulation and inhibition of cell proliferation: New mechanistic insights. *Cell* 63, 245-247.

Nakatsukasa, H., Evarts, R.P., Hsia, C-C. and Thorgeirsson, S.S. (1990): Transforming growth factor β1 and Type 1 procollagen transcripts during regeneration and early fibrosis of rat liver. *Lab. Invest.* 63, 171-180.

Noguchi, S., Ohba, Y. and Oka, T. (1991): Influence of epidermal growth factor on liver regeneration after partial hepatectomy in mice. *J. Endocrinol.* 128, 425-431.

Noguchi, S., Ohba, Y. and Oka, T. (1992): The role of transcription and messenger RNA stability in the regulation of epidermal growth factor receptor gene expression in regenerating mouse liver. *Hepatology* 15, 88-96.

Olsen, P.S., Boesby, S., Kirkegaard, P. Therkelsen, K., Almdal, T., Poulsen, S.S. and Nexϕ, E. (1988): Influence of epidermal growth factor on liver regeneration after partial hepatectomy in rats. *Hepatology* 8, 992-996.

Rall, L.B., Scott, J. and Bell, G.I. (1985): Mouse prepro-epidermal growth factor synthesis by the kidney and other tissues. *Nature* 313, 228-231.

Roberts, A.B. and Sporn, M.B. (1985): Transforming growth factors. *Cancer Surveys* 4, 683-705.

Roberts, A.B., Anzano, M.A., Wakefield, L.M., Roche, N.S., Stern, D.F. and Sporn, M.B. (1985): Type beta transforming growth factor: a bifunctional regulator of cellular growth. *Proc. Natl. Acad. Sci. U.S.A.* 82, 119-123.

Roberts, A.B. and Sporn, M.B. (1989): The transforming growth factor-βs. In *Peptide growth factors and their receptors*, ed. M.B. Sporn and A.B. Roberts, pp. 419-472. Handbook of experimental pharmacology, vol 95. Berlin: Springer-Verlag.

Sandgren, E.P, Luetteke, N.C., Palmiter, R.D., Brinster, R.L. and Lee, D.C. (1990): Overexpression of TGFα in transgenic mice induces liver neoplasia and abnormal development of the mammary gland and pancreas. *Cell* 61, 1137-1146.

Winkler, M.E., O'Connor, L., Winget, M. and Fendly, B. (1989): Epidermal growth factor and transforming growth factor α bind differently to the epidermal growth factor receptor. *Biochemistry* 28, 6373-6378.

Yeh, Y-C., Tsai, J-F., Chuang, L-Y., Yeh, H-W., Tsai, J-H., Florine, D.L. and Tam, J.P. (1987): Elevation of transforming growth factor α and its relationship to the epidermal growth factor and α-fetoprotein levels in patients with hepatocellular carcinoma. *Cancer Res.* 47, 896-901.

Liver Regeneration. Eds D. Bernuau, G. Feldmann. John Libbey Eurotext, Paris © 1992, pp. 85-101.

Hepatocyte growth factor (HGF)

George K. Michalopoulos, Reza Zarnegar, Ranugath Appasamy

University of Pittsburgh, School of Medicine, Pittsburgh, PA 15261, USA

Adapted from Michalopoulos, GK, Zarnegar, R. Hepatocyte Growth Factor. Hepatology, 1992; 15:149-155, with permission from Mosby-Year Book, Inc.

Introduction and History of Discovery

Early studies had suggested that factors circulating in the blood during liver regeneration after 2/3 partial hepatectomy stimulate hepatic proliferation in livers of parabiotic circulation partners (Moolten et al., 1967; Fisher et al., 1970) grafted hepatic tissue (Grisham et al., 1964) or transplanted isolated hepatocytes (Jirtle & Michalopoulos, 1982). Subsequent studies from our laboratory (Michalopoulos et al. 1983; Michalopoulos et al., 1984) demonstrated the existence of a growth factor in the large molecular weight fraction of the plasma which stimulated growth of hepatocytes in primary culture. This was the main detectable polypeptide mitogenic activity that could be identified in the plasma over the whole range of molecular weights. A smaller glycolipid with weaker mitogenic activity was also identified and called Hepatopoietin B (Michalopoulos et al., 1984). The large molecular weight factor was initially called Hepatopoietin A (Michalopoulos et al., 1983; Michalopoulos et al., 1984) or Hepatotropin (Nakamura et al., 1984). A similar activity had also been found previously in rat platelets (Russell et al., 1984). This factor was isolated in three separate laboratories and from diverse plasma sources by heparin affinity chromatography and reverse phase high pressure liquid chromatography (Nakamura et al., 1987; Gohda et al., 1988; Zarnegar et al., 1989). Despite its apparent molecular weight of 200 - 300 kD in molecular sieve chromatography (Zarnegar et al., 1989), separation by HPLC revealed that the active mitogenic principle had a molecular weight closer to 100 kD (Nakamura et al., 1987; Gohda et al., 1988; Zarnegar et al., 1989). The difference in apparent molecular weights suggests that the form of HGF circulating in the plasma may be bound to a carrier molecule. The molecule consisted of two chains (70 and 30 kD respectively) which were dissociable in reducing gel electrophoresis (Nakamura et al., 1987; Gohda et al., 1988; Zarnegar et al., 1989).

A partial amino acid sequence for rabbit Hepatopoietin A (Zarnegar et al., 1989) and a complete amino acid sequence for human HGF deduced from cloning the entire cDNA from a human placenta library (Miyazawa et al., 1989) showed that the entities were the same. A confirming paper with the entire sequence of HGF from human liver also soon appeared, showing essentially an identical sequence with minor differences (Nakamura et al., 1989). The latter publication also described the secondary structure of HGF and and the presence of kringles. The small differences in sequence between the two groups were reconciled in a subsequent publication (Seki et al., 1990) confirming as correct the sequence identified from human placenta.

After the primary structure of HGF cDNA was identified, molecular cloning of the cDNA for an entity known as Scatter Factor showed that it was identical to HGF (Seki et al., 1990). A recent detail paper on this issue confirmed the identity of HGF and Scatter Factor and showed that they are encoded from a single gene (Weidner et al., 1991). Molecular cloning of another entity known as Tumor Cytotoxic Factor also demonstrated that it was identical to HGF (Higashio et al., 1990). For the effects of these molecules and the broader implications for the function of HGF in tissues see below.

HGF structure: The deduced amino acid sequence of HGF revealed a substantial homology to plasminogen and a very interesting structure (Nakamura et al., 1989; Michalopoulos, 1990). The heavy chain of HGF (called alpha chain) consists of four kringle domains similar to the kringle domains described for other proteins. Kringles are double loop polypeptide structures in which a smaller loop is held together with disulfide bonds within a larger loop. A characteristic sequence (NYCRNP) is present in all kringles in a characteristic location. The kringle domains present in HGF have substantial sequence homology to kringle domains 1, 4, 5 of plasminogen and to kringle 1 of prothrombin. Several functions have been assigned to kringles in other proteins, in general related to the abilities of kringle bearing proteins to bind or intercalate with other proteins. The light chain of HGF (called beta chain) has the structure of a pseudo-protease (of the serine protease superfamily). In functioning serine proteases, the amino acids serine, histidine and aspartate come in close three dimensional proximity to form the catalytic site for the protease. Consensus sequences common in all serine proteases surround each of the amino acids which form the catalytic site. The beta chain of HGF has preserved most of the consensus sequences found in this class of proteases. Two of the three amino acids forming the catalytic site, however, have been altered (serine into tyrosine and histidine into glutamine). All studies performed so far have failed to reveal any protease function for HGF.

The structure of HGF is most unusual for a growth factor. The presence of kringles and the pseudo-protease domain suggests recent phylogenetic derivation. Its distribution in the phylogenetic tree, however, has not been yet determined. Homologies are seen with several proteins, especially proteins bearing kringles. Many plasma proteins and coagulation associated proteins fall in this category. Strong homologies in amino acid sequence exist between HGF and other kringle bearing proteins such as plasminogen (31%), tissue plasminogen activator, factor XII, etc. Strong homologies are also present between the beta chain of HGF and serine proteases such as kalikrein, factor XI etc.
Molecular processing: The native form of HGF is synthesized as a single chain precursor, consisting of 728 amino acids. (Miyazawa et al., 1989; Nakamura et al., 1989; Okajima et al., 1990). The N-terminal amino acid of the precursor molecule is pyroglutamate, derived from glutamine at the 32nd residue from the initiation site encoding methionine (Yoshiyama et al., 1991). HGF is extracted from a variety of sources as a mixture of

single chain precursor and a two chain heterodimer (Hernandez et al., in press; Rubin et al., 1991). Both biologic forms appear equally active (Hernandez et al., in press). The two chain heterodimer consists of a heavy (alpha) chain and a light (beta) chain. The heterodimer is derived by cleavage of the single chain form next to arginine (in position 494) and prior to valine (position 495). The cleavage site arg-val-val is the same as the one resulting in activation of plasminogen to plasmin by tissue plasminogen activator (TPA). This suggests that TPA may indeed be the natural enzyme causing the conversion of the the single-chain HGF to the heterodimeric form (Rubin et al., 1991). This, however, has not been directly confirmed. If this were to be true, it would be quite interesting, given the dramatic increase of TPA in most neoplasms. The increase of TPA seen in neoplasia may locally mediate the activation of HGF and result in enhanced migration and/mitogenesis of epithelial cells (Rubin et al., 1991) (see Scatter Factor effects, below). Attractive as this hypothesis may be it remains to be proven directly. As mentioned above, the single chain HGF is biologically active (Hernandez et al., in press). This can imply that activation to the heterodimeric form is not required for biologic activity or that the enzymes causing the conversion to heterodimeric form are so ubiquitous that they are not rate limiting.

Smaller forms of HGF were recently described, consisting of a variant of 28 kD (Bottaro et al., 1991) with receptor binding properties similar to that of HGF. This may result from a recently described alternate pathway for HGF mRNA splicing, resulting in molecule consisting of the first 290 amino acids of the heavy chain. The latter molecule however did not have biologic activity in hepatocyte cultures (Miyazawa et al., 1991). Multiple forms of mRNA cross-hybridizing with various HGF derived probes are seen in hepatocytes during liver regeneration (Zarnegar et al., 1991). Whether these forms of mRNA represent true alternate splicing variants translated into proteins with biologic functions or whether they are non-translatable mRNAs remains to be further determined.

The structure of HGF gene was recently described (Seki et al., 1991). The gene has features of overall organization akin to those of other coagulation associated proteases. It is composed of 18 exons separated by 17 introns and it spans approximately 70 kb. As with other kringle containing proteins, each kringle is encoded by two exons. Recent studies have localized the HGF gene on human chromosome 7 (Weidner et al., 1991; Zarnegar et al., in press). (Note: c-met, the gene encoding the receptor for HGF, is also localized on the same chromosome, in close proximity).

Sources of HGF. HGF is present in measurable amounts in plasma (Michalopoulos et al., 1984; Gohda et al., 1988). Increased amounts of HGF present in serum led to isolation of HGF from platelets (Nakamura et al., 1984; Russell et al., 1984). The first reported cloning of the HGF cDNA was derived from a placental cDNA library (Miyazawa et al., 1989). HGF mRNA was found in Northern blots from from adult rat lung, kidney, brain, liver, thymus and submandibular gland (Tashiro et al., 1990). HGF mRNA was also found in human fetal liver (Selden et al., 1990), placenta (Miyazawa et al., 1989), and embryonic lung fibroblasts (Rubin et al., 1991). In situ hybridization studies have been carried in liver. Past studies localized HGF mRNA in non-parenchymal cells (Noji et al., 1990). A recent study by Schirmacher (Schirmacher et al., 1992) shows conclusively that the main cell type producing HGF in liver is the cell of Ito. A recent previous study from our laboratory also showed that the primary site of HGF localization in normal rat liver was in non-parenchymal cells (Wolf et al., 1991).

Although our study identified these cells as endothelial and Kupffer cells, the studies presented by Schirmacher (Schirmacher et al., 1992) clearly show that the cell types we described probably included or likely were in their majority Ito cells. Given the fact that we did not use any histochemical stains to further identify the non-parenchymal cell types that we described and the fact that Ito cells are difficult to characterize in tissue sections in the absence of special stains, this is the most likely explanation. Other previous studies using in situ hybridization, however, have also identified endothelial cells and Kupffer cells as the sources of HGF in normal and damaged livers (Noji et al., 1990). The studies presented in ref. 65 are the only one in which the cell types were isolated as homogeneous populations and in which HGF mRNA could be identified by Northern gel. Thus these studies are the most convincing. Based on these studies, Ito cells appear to be the main type producing HGF mRNA in normal liver.

HGF protein was also localized in several other tissues using HGF specific antibodies (Wolf et al., 1991). In liver, as mentioned above, HGF protein was localized in non-parenchymal cell types. HGF protein was not found in hepatocytes from normal or regenerating liver. HGF was seen in hepatocytes damaged by carbon tetrachloride (Lindroos et al., 1991). The in situ hybridization data mentioned above (Noji et al., 1990) strongly suggest that presence of HGF in damaged hepatocytes is a result of passive uptake from other HGF producing cell types (Ito cells and invading macrophages).

Of equal interest to its localization in the liver is the presence of HGF protein in several cell types in other tissues. HGF protein was localized in tissues in which HGF mRNA has been found and in several additional tissues (Wolf et al., 1991). The histochemical localization in some tissues was confirmed by extraction and antibody neutralization of the extracted HGF from these tissues (Zarnegar et al., 1990). In the central nervous system, HGF was found in large neurons of brain cortex and cerebellum and motor neurons of the spinal cord. In normal placenta, HGF was localized in the syncytiotrophoblast, with cytotrophoblast being negative (Wolf et al., 1991). HGF was found in the cytotrophoblast cells however in hydatidiform moles and choriocarcinoma (Wolf et al., 1991). HGF was also found throughout the gastrointestinal mucosa, in all squamous epithelia (including uterine cervix and Hassal's corpuscles of the thymus), and in all lining glandular epithelia, including breast ducts, tracheobronchial columnar epithelium, prostate glands etc. (Wolf et al., 1991). Human ovum also appeared to contain HGF protein. In the kidney, HGF was found primarily in the distal tubules and collecting ducts. Strong immunoreactivity was seen in the cells of exocrine pancreas. The latter is of interest because HGF mRNA was not found in pancreas in previous studies (Tashiro et al., 1990). The absence of HGF mRNA in pancreas, however, may be due to the notorious difficulty in isolation of intact mRNA from pancreas, due to high concentrations of ribonuclease. The presence of HGF in many tissues feeding into the portal circulation suggests that trophic effects for the liver through the portal circulation may be exercised through HGF from sites other than intrahepatic. HGF was also localized in several embryonic tissues, in general similar to those seen in adult animals (DeFrances et al., unpublished observations).

Though there is overall good correspondence between presence of HGF mRNA in several tissues and localization of HGF protein in cells from these tissues, it remains to be seen whether HGF protein is actually produced or merely taken up by the cells in which it is localized by specific immunohistochemistry. HGF has so far found to be produced only by mesenchymal cell lines in culture (Weidner et al., 1991; Rubin et al., 1991). If HGF is produced only be mesenchymal cells but heavily localized in epithelial cells it may be a very important contributor for the variously documented trophic interactions between mesenchymal and parenchymal cells in many tissues.

Effects of HGF on different cell types.

Mitogenic effects: Given the fact that HGF was isolated using the bioassay of stimulation of DNA synthesis in primary cultures of hepatocytes, the effects of HGF on hepatocytes are the best characterized. HGF is mitogenic for rat (Nakamura et al., 1984; Russell et al., 1984; Nakamura et al., 1987; Gohda et al., 1988; Zarnegar et al., 1989; Hernadez et al., in press) and human (Strain et al., 1991) hepatocytes maintained in serum free, chemically defined, media and in the absence of other mitogenic factors. The effect is seen in doses as small as 1 ng/ml, with a maximal effect seen in the range of 5-10 ng/ml. On a molar basis, HGF is the most potent mitogen for hepatocytes. The nuclear labeling index reaches 75%-80%. The effect of HGF is inhibited by TGF, partially inhibited by heparin (Zarnegar et al., 1989) and enhanced by the comitogen norepinephrine (Lindroos et al., 1991). Additive effects are seen between HGF and EGF. Hepatocytes phenotypically stabilizd with 2% DMSO do not respond to HGF or the other two hepatocyte peptide mitogens (EGF and aFGF) (Kost et al., 1991). Prompt response to HGF is seen as soon as DMSO is removed. HGF also stimulates DNA synthesis in hepatocytes in vivo when injected into the portal vein of the dog (Francavilla et al., in press). In addition to DNA synthesis, HGF also stimulates protein synthesis in hepatocytes (Hernandez et al., in press). This effect is not substantially inhibited by TGF. In addition to mitogenic effects on hepatocytes, several recent papers (Rubin et al., 1991; Kan et al., 1991; Matsumoto et al., 1991; Igawa et al., 1991;) describe mitogenic effects of HGF on other cell types. HGF stimulates DNA synthesis in renal proximal tubular epithelial cells, melanocytes, keratinocytes (Kan et al., 1991), breast carcinoma and melanoma cells kidney epithelial cells transformed by SV40. HGF did not stimulate DNA synthesis in fibroblasts. The effects of HGF on hepatoma cells have not been fully characterized. Some of the hepatoma cell lines tested (i.e. H3B) do not respond to HGF. The effects on tubular epithelium are additive with EGF and aFGF and inhibited by TGF. The effects on melanocytes are also inhibited by TGF.

Effects on cell motility.
Literature from the work on Scatter Factor (subsequently identified as HGF, as mentioned above) has documented several effects of HGF on cell motility. Several epithelial and endothelial cell lines "scatter" upon addition of HGF to the medium. The scattering effect is best summarized as cell dissociation and migration and it is precisely measured in specific assays. The effect is seen in variable concentrations. The concentrations causing scattering effects and mitogenic effects do not always coincide and it has been stated that HGF exercises only scattering effects in some cell lines in the absence of mitogenic activity (Rosen et al., 1989; Stoker et al., 1987). This is a very important issue raising questions about the number of receptors involved in HGF effects and the multiplicity of signal transduction pathways for the HGF receptor(s). As mentioned above, scattering effects are induced only on epithelial and endothelial cells but not on fibroblasts or mesenchymal cells. It should also be mentioned that HGF has both mitogenic and "scattering" effects on hepatocytes in identical concentrations (Nakamura et al., 1984; Russell et al., 1984; Nakamura et al., 1987; Gohda et all., 1988; Zarnegar et al., 1989; Hernandez et al., in press). Addition of HGF in hepatocyte

cultures induces formation of long processes and cell migration. These morphologic changes appear before and during DNA synthesis and are much more pronounced than similar changes induced by EGF.

Tumor cytotoxic effects. High concentrations of HGF induce inhibit growth or are cytotoxic to some carcinoma and sarcoma cell lines (Higashio et al., 1990). The mechanism for this effect and the reason for the high concentrations required is not very clear.

HGF receptor. Independent studies from two laboratories (Bottaro et al., 1991; Naldini et al., 1991) have shown conclusively that the protein encoded by the proto-oncogene known as c-met is a receptor for HGF. This oncogene encodes for a protein of a molecular weight of 190 kD. It is composed of two chains (alpha chain: 145 kD and beta chain: 50 kD) combined in a heterodimeric form by disulfide bonds. The protein has the configuration of a type II tyrosine kinase receptor, with extracellular binding domains, transmembrane portions and intra-cytosolic protein kinase domain (Giordano, et al., 1989). Addition of nanomolar concentrations of HGF to a gastric carcinoma cell line with amplified c-met enhanced the phosphorylation on tyrosine of the p190c-met kinase. Addition of other known growth factors or serum was ineffective. The kinase activity of the c-MET receptor was also stimulated by HGF in an in vitro assay, after detergent solubilization and partial purification of p190c-met. The specific activation of the tyrosine kinase function of the met protein by nanomolar concentrations of HGF and the subsequent demonstration of crosslinking between whole HGF and c-met after mixing purified preparations clearly show that met protein is a receptor for HGF. The HGF receptor encoded by c-met is distributed in many tissues, including liver, skin, uterus, brain, lungs, kidney, etc. (Naldini et al., 1991). The widespread distribution of the met protein demonstrates the importance of HGF not only for liver regeneration but for growth and differentiation in many other tissues. It remains to be seen whether met protein is the only receptor for HGF. As mentioned above, several findings such as loss of mitogenic effects or acquisition of mito-inhibitory and cytotoxic properties at high concentrations, as well as the apparent dissociation between "scattering" effects and mitogenic effects for some cell lines raise the issue that the met protein may not be the only receptor for HGF. On the other hand, the mode of action of met is not clearly understood. Better delineation of the signal transduction pathways stimulated by met may provide explanations for these discrepancies and reconcile the existing contradictory data with a single receptor model. Direct studies of binding of HGF on hepatocytes have shown high affinity binding sites variably estimated from 1000 (Higuchi et al., 1991) to 120,000 (Zarnegar et al., 1990) sites per hepatocyte. Lower affinity sites were also detected in higher (Zarnegar et al., 1990) numbers. The latter might be of importance for the mito-inhibitory effects seen at large HGF concentrations.

HGF and Liver regeneration. The early findings showing that HGF is the only protein mitogen for hepatocytes present in the plasma (Michalopoulos et al., 1983; Michalopoulos et al., 1984) make HGF the most likely candidate for the cross-circulating mitogen stimulating proliferation of hepatocytes in non-hepatectomized parabiotic circulation partners of hepatectomized rats and in grafted hepatic tissue and transplanted isolated hepatocytes in extrahepatic sites (Moolten et al., 1967; Fisher et al., 1970;

Grisham et al., 1964; Jirtle et al., 1982). More recent studies (Lindroos et al., 1991) have measured the changes in HGF levels in plasma after 2/3 partial hepatectomy in rats or after carbon tetrachloride intoxication and have reinforced the crucial role for HGF in liver regeneration. These findings are as follows:

1. HGF levels rise in the plasma 15-17 fold within 1-2 hours after 2/3 partial hepatectomy, reaching concentrations which are well above the mitogenic range for hepatocytes in culture. The levels return to lower values within 24 hours. DNA synthesis ensues with a peak at 24 hours (Lindroos et al., 1991)
2. HGF levels also rise very shortly after carbon tetrachloride intoxication and remain elevated for 24-36 hours. DNA synthesis ensues with a peak at 48 hours after intoxication (Lindroos et al., 1991).
3. HGF mRNA in rat liver increases within 3-6 hours after 2/3 partial hepatectomy, peaks at 20 hours and returns to basal levels by 72 hours. (Zarnegar et al., 1991; Kinoshita et al., 1991).
4. Injection of HGF directly into the portal vein led to DNA synthesis in the liver of dogs. (Francavilla et al., in press)

The early steep increase of HGF levels in the plasma following 2/3 partial hepatectomy and preceding by many hours the initiation of DNA synthesis, makes HGF the best candidate for triggering the multiple effects described following 2/3 partial hepatectomy. Its rise within 1 hour is consistent with the early changes in gene expression in liver seen within 30 minutes after 2/3 partial hepatectomy. The mechanism for the rise is not clear at this point. The elevation of HGF protein in the plasma prior to the elevation of HGF mRNA in the liver clearly suggests that HGF increase in the plasma is not due to increased synthesis from hepatic sources. Though platelets contain large amounts of HGF, induction of severe thrombocytopenia in rats did not interfere with liver regeneration, suggesting that platelets are not involved with the generation of any relevant mitogenic signals for this process (Kuwashima et al., 1990). Given the wide tissue distribution of HGF, it is conceivable that HGF is released in the plasma from a variety of sources. If circulating HGF is normally cleared by liver, acute reduction in liver mass (following hepatic resection) or loss of the capacity to clear HGF (following toxins) may explain the acute rise of HGF prior to DNA synthesis. Recent studies in our laboratory (Appasamy et al., unpublished observations) demonstrate that in fact liver is the major organ involved in clearance of HGF. Injection of radioactive labeled HGF shows that liver sequesters by far the largest amount of HGF compared to any other organ. More than 40% of the injected HGF is rapidly sequestered in the liver. Radioactivity associated with HGF or its degradation products appears in the bile 5 minutes after injection. The half life of HGF and the plasma clearance are dramatically affected by 2/3 partial hepatectomy. The decrease in HGF plasma clearance seen shortly after hepatectomy is consistent with our hypothesis that diminished plasma clearance of HGF is the reason for the HGF elevation in the plasma following 2/3 partial hepatectomy. Such acute elevation of plasma values is also known to occur for norepinephrine. Norepinephrine amplifies the mitogenic effect of HGF and EGF on hepatocytes (Lindroos et al., 1991). Its rise in the plasma after 2/3 partial hepatectomy follows similar kinetics with the rise of HGF (Cruise et al., 1987). Since circulating

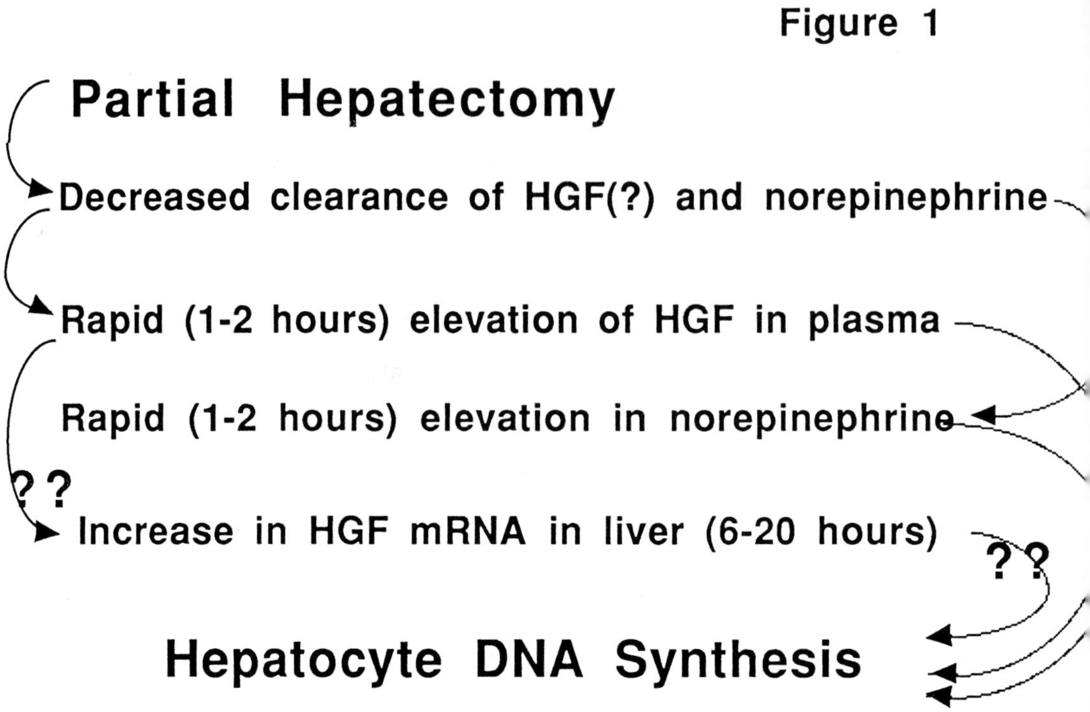

Figure 1

Partial Hepatectomy

Decreased clearance of HGF(?) and norepinephrine

Rapid (1-2 hours) elevation of HGF in plasma

Rapid (1-2 hours) elevation in norepinephrine

?? Increase in HGF mRNA in liver (6-20 hours) ??

Hepatocyte DNA Synthesis

Figure 1: Proposed scheme for the role of HGF in stimulating DNA synthesis in hepatocytes after 2/3 partial hepatectomy. Steps not as yet proven are marked with double question marks. The curved arrows indicate the cause and effect relationship between the different steps.

norepinephrine is known to be degraded by the hepatic monoamine oxidase, removal of 2/3 of the liver results in dramatic decrease in capacity to degrade norepinephrine resulting in increased concentration in the plasma. Norepinephrine is one of the strongest co-mitogens for hepatocytes in culture. We have proposed (Lindroos et al., 1991) that the simultaneous elevation of HGF and norepinephrine very shortly after partial hepatectomy provides the mitotic stimulus leading to liver regeneration. A proposed scheme to integrate the above findings for HGF and liver regeneration is shown in Figure 1.

The above findings are important in that they provide evidence for the first time for the emergence of a mitogenic signal for the liver which precedes hepatocyte DNA synthesis. Recent studies from other laboratories have shown that regenerating hepatocytes produce TGFa (Mead et al., 1989) and aFGF (Kan et al., 1989). This has led to the hypothesis that liver regeneration is driven by autocrine growth factors. According to this hypothesis, hepatocytes become primed by metabolic signals, following which they move from G_0 to G_1 phase of the cell cycle and start producing autocrine growth factors (TGFa and aFGF). This leads to hepatocyte DNA synthesis. The major drawback of this model is that the above growth factors are produced by the regenerating hepatocytes at the time of DNA synthesis and not prior to the DNA synthesis. HGF and norepinephrine in the plasma, on the other hand, are at their peak levels many hours prior to the initiation of DNA synthesis. This should not imply that production of TGFa and aFGF by regenerating hepatocytes is not important. Given the time relationship between emergence of the growth factor and initiation of DNA synthesis, it does not appear that TGFa and aFGF are the major stimuli leading to first wave of hepatocyte DNA synthesis. It is likely, on the other hand, that these factors may influence the second and third wave of hepatocyte mitogenesis. It is also likely that these factors have an "angiogenic" role. Following partial hepatectomy, DNA synthesis in hepatic endothelial cells is seen almost precisely 24 hours after the peak of DNA synthesis in hepatocytes (Grisham et al., 1962). Thus the production of aFGF and TGFa may be responsible not for autocrine stimulation of hepatocytes but for a paracrine stimulation of DNA synthesis in endothelial cells. The rise of HGF mRNA in the liver following rise of HGF in the plasma may also contribute to hepatocyte mitogenesis by paracrine release of HGF or it may a role specific to the function of the mRNA producing cells.

The sharp changes in HGF concentrations in the plasma following 2/3 partial hepatectomy or during hepatic failure recently reported by Tomiya (Tomiya et al., 1992) suggest the possibility that HGF production and release by several tissues may have an endocrine role for the liver. Paracrine effects might also be of importance via HGF produced by the cells of Ito (Schirmacher et al., 1992).

If HGF rise in the plasma is the major drive for hepatic regeneration, and given the fact that HGF stimulates DNA synthesis of many several cell types, why is regeneration limited to the liver and not to other organs? Currently there is no clear answer to this question. It should be noted, however, that 2/3 partial hepatectomy leads to DNA synthesis not only in the liver but also in the exocrine portion of the pancreas (Rao & Subbarao, 1986). Enhanced expression of cell cycle related genes (c-Ha-ras and c-myc) was also seen in the kidney following 2/3 partial hepatectomy, though this was not followed by DNA synthesis. (Roesel et al., 1989). Such studies have not been carried by other tissues. The above findings suggest that the rise of HGF in the plasma after 2/3 partial hepatectomy causes effects in other target tissues. The limitation of the mitogenic effects to the liver may be due to specific regulatory pathways particular to these tissues. It is also possible that the specificity of response to the high levels of HGF in the plasma may be controlled by co-mitogens (in this instance, norepinephrine).

HGF and liver disease. One of the original sources for isolation of HGF was plasma of patients with fulminant hepatitis (Gohda et al., 1988). Subsequent studies by the same laboratory (Gohda et al., 1991; Tsubouchi et al., 1991; Tsubouchi et al., 1991; Gohda et al., 1990) have well documented that HGF rises to extremely high levels in the plasma of these patients. The reason for the rise in HGF levels is not clear. It is well documented, however, that acute fulminant hepatitis is associated with dramatic decrease in numbers of parenchymal hepatocytes, leading in some cases to complete elimination of the parenchymal cells from the liver (acute yellow atrophy). Thus, the reason for the elevation of HGF in this condition may be similar to the reasons leading to rise of HGF when 2/3 of the liver tissue is resected. It was also recently shown that HGF rises in the plasma during acute (non-fulminant) hepatitis (Tsubouchi et al., 1991), though the levels were much less and not as consistent as with fulminant hepatitis. Increased levels of HGF were also found in ascites from patients with cirrhosis (Shimizu, et al., 1991). Additional very interesting results on changes of HGF plasma levels in liver disease and chronic renal failure were recently presented by Tomiya et al. using a sensitive ELISA kit newly available for HGF (Tomiya et al., 1992). These and the above findings underscore the correlation between HGF and chronic liver disease. In view of the high levels of HGF in many cases of cirrhosis as documented by Tomiya et al., it is unlikely that there is a decrease in HGF available to hepatocytes during cirrhosis, as postulated by Schirmacher (Schirmacher et al., 1992). In fact, there is an overall increase in proliferative activity in most types of cirrhosis and this may correlate with the findings by Tomiya (Tomiya et al., 1992). The increase in HGF levels after hemodialysis is puzzling but it may be due to "extraction" of tissue bound HGF by the anti-coagulant heparin (Nasyniti et al., 1991). Either way, the findings from this and the previously referred manuscripts clearly document that fulminant hepatic failure is not due to lack of available circulating HGF. The production of HGF by Ito cells in fulminant hepatitis should also be assessed.

Also of interest is the finding by Tomiya et al. of elevation of HGF in chronic kidney failure (1a). As mentioned above, HGF stimulated proliferation of proximal tubular cells while been localized to the collecting ductules (Wolf et al., 1991; Kan et al., 1991; Igawa et al., 1991). Correlations between levels of HGF and proliferation of kidney cell populations need to be made in order to better understand the significance of these findings.

HGF: Current puzzles and future studies: Given the fact that HGF was only isolated, cloned and sequenced less than three years ago, the accumulated information on HGF and its biologic functions is appreciable. More knowledge, however, needs to be gained. Clearly, HGF is bound to have a role in embryonic development (Stern et al., 1990), as well as in other phenomena dependent on cell migration, such as tumor invasion and metastasis. Its presence in high levels in placenta, brain, lungs, and so many other tissues, suggests that it plays a fundamental role in function of many cell types. If HGF is produced only by mesenchymal cells but sequestered and active only on parenchymal and epithelial cells, it may be a very important factor for mesenchymal-parenchymal cell interactions. Another potential target of studies may be the effect of long term elevations in plasma HGF during chronic liver disease for other tissues sensitive to its effects. Such tissues should definitely include kidney and pancreas, in which DNA synthesis or entry into G_1 is seen after partial hepatectomy. It should also include other tissues in which the met protein is present, such as brain, gastrointestinal mucosa, skin etc. Clearly, future studies on mechanisms of liver cell proliferation and chronic liver disease cannot be complete in the absence of a context related to HGF levels and HGF effects. In that sense, HGF is here to stay as far as hepatic biology is concerned. For many of us this is a welcome change. In the pantheon of GFs, an important prefix letter missing was H. Now Hepar has its growth factor, though it clearly has to share it with other tissues, as was the case in the past with epidermis (EGF), fibroblasts (FGF) etc. This, however, is only an anthropomorphic problem. Tissues know better.

REFERENCES

Appasamy, R., Zarnegar, R., and Michalopoulos, G.K. Unpublished observations.

Bottaro, D.P., Rubin, J.S., D.L., Chan, A.M., Kmiecik, T.E., Vande Woude G.F., Aaronson, S.A. (1991): Identification of the hepatocyte growth factor receptor as the c-met proto-oncogene product. Science 251:802-804.

Cruise, J.L., Knechtle, S., Bollinger, R.R., Kuhn, C., and Michalopoulos, G. (1987): Alpha-1 adrenergic effects and liver regeneration. Hepatology, 7:1189-1194.

DeFrances, M., Michalopoulos, G.K., Wolf, H., Zarnegar, R. Unpublished observations.

Fisher, B., Szuch, P., Levine, M., and Fisher, E. (1970): A Portal Blood Factor as the Humoral Agent in Liver Regeneration. Science 171:575-577.

Francavilla, A., Starzl, T.E., Porter, K., Scotti-Foglieni, C., Michalopoulos, G.K., Carrieri, G., Trejo, J., Azzarone, A., Barone, M., Zeng, Q. Screening for candidate hepatic growth factors by selective portal infusion after canine Eck fistula. Hepatology, In Press.

Gherardi, E., and Stoker, M. (1990): Hepatocytes and scatter factor [letter] Nature Jul 19;346(6281):228

Giordano, S., Ponzetto, C., Di Renzo, M.F., Cooper, C.S., and Comoglio, P.M. Tyrosine kinase receptor indistinguishable from the c-met protein. (1989): Nature 339:155-156.

Gohda, E., Tusubouchi, H., Nakayama, H., Hirono, S., Sakiyama, O., Takahashi, K., Miyazaki H. (1988): Purification and Partial Characterization of Hepatocyte Growth Factor from Plasma of a Patient with Fulminant Hepatic Failure. J. Clin. Invest. 81:414-419.

Gohda, E., Tsubouchi, H., Nakayama, H., Hirono, S., Arakaki, N., Yamamoto, I, Hashimoto, S., and Daikuhara, Y. (1991): Human hepatocyte growth factor in blood of patients with fulminant hepatic failure. Basic Aspects. Dig Dis Sci; 36:785-790.

Gohda, E., Yamasaki, T., Tsubouchi, H., Kurobe, M., Sakiyama, O., Aoki, H., Niidani N., Shin, S., Hayashi, K., Hashimoto, S, et al. (1990): Biological and immunological properties of human hepatocyte growth factor from plasma of patients with fulminant hepatic failure. Biochim Biophys Acta 1053:21-26.

Grisham, J.W., Leong, G.F., and Hole, B.V. (1964): Heterotopic partial autotransplantation of rat liver. Technique and demonstration of structure and function of the graft. Cancer Res. 24:1474-1482.

Hernandez, J., Zarnegar, R., and Michalopoulos, G.K. Characterization of the effects of human placental HGF on rat hepatocytes. J. Cell Phys., In Press.

Higashio, K., Shima, N., Goto, M., Itagaki, Y., Nagao, M., Yasuda, H., et al., (1990): Identity of a tumor cytotoxic factor from human fibroblasts and hepatocyte growth factor. Biochem. Biophys. Res. Commun. 170(1):397-404.

Higuchi, O., and Nakamura, T. (1991): Identification and change in the receptor for hepatocyte growth factor in rat liver after partial hepatectomy or induced hepatitis. Biochem. Biophys. Res. Commun. 176:599-607.

Igawa, T., Kanda, S., Kanetake, H., Saitoh, Y., Ichihara, A., Tomita, Y., et al. (1991): Hepatocyte growth factor is a potent mitogen for cultured rabbit renal tubular epithelial cells. Biochem. Biophys. Res. Commun. 174(2):831-838.

Jirtle, R.L., and Michalopoulos, G. (1982): Effects of partial hepatectomy on transplanted hepatocytes. Cancer Res. 42:3000-3004.

Kan, M., Huan, J., Mansson, P., Yasumitsu, H., Carr, B., and McKeehan, W. (1989): Heparin-binding growth factor type 1 (acidic fibroblast growth factor): A potential biphasic autocrine and paracrine regulator of hepatocyte regeneration. Proc. Nat. Acad. Sci. (USA), 86:7432-7436.

Kan, M., Zhang, G.H., Zarnegar, R., Michalopoulos, G., Myoken, Y., McKeehan, et al. (1991): JI Hepatocyte growth factor/hepatopoietin A stimulates the growth of rat kidney proximal tubule epithelial cells (RPTE), rat nonparenchymal liver cells, human melanoma cells, mouse keratinocytes and stimulates anchorage-independent growth of SV-40 transformed RPTE. Biochem. Biophys. Res. Commun. 174:331-337.

Kinoshita, T., Hirao, S., Matsumoto, K., and Nakamura, T. (1991): Possible endocrine control by hepatocyte growth factor of liver regeneration after partial hepatectomy. Biochem. Biophys. Res. Commun. 177:330-335.

Kost, D.P., and Michalopoulos, G.K. (1991): Effect of 2% dimethyl sulfoxide on the mitogenic properties of epidermal growth factor and hepatocyte growth factor in primary hepatocyte culture. J. Cell. Physiol. 147:274-280.

Kuwashima, Y., Aoki, K., Kohyyama, K., and Ishikawa, T. (1990): Hepatocyte Regeneration after partial hepatectomy occurs even under several thrombocytopenic conditions in the rat. Jpn. J. Cancer Res. 81:607-612.

Lindroos, P.M., Zarnegar, R., and Michalopoulos, G.K. (1991): Hepatic Growth Factor (Hepatopoietin A) Rapidly Increases in Plasma Prior to DNA Synthesis and Liver Regeneration Stimulated by Partial Hepatectomy and CCl4 Administration. Hepatology 13:743-750.

Masumoto, A., and Yamamoto, N. (1991): Sequestration of a hepatocyte growth factor in extracellular matrix in normal adult rat liver. Biochem. Biophys. Res. Commun. 174:90-95.

Matsumoto, K., Tajima, H., and Nakamura, T. (1991): Hepatocyte growth factor is a potent stimulator of human melanocyte DNA synthesis and growth. Biochem. Biophys. Res. Commun. 176:45-51.

Mead, J.E., and Fausto, N. (1989): Transforming growth factor TGFa may be a physiological regulator of liver regeneration by means of an autocrine mechanism. Proc. Natl. Acad. Sci. USA, 86:1558-1562.

Michalopoulos, G.K. (1990): Liver regeneration: Molecular Mechanisms of growth control. F.A.S.E.B. Journal 4:240-249.

Michalopoulos, G., Houck, K.A., Dolan, M.L., and Luetteke, N.C. (1984): Control of hepatocyte proliferation by two serum factors. Cancer Res. 44:4414-4419.

Michalopoulos, G., Houck, K., Dolan, M., and Novicki, D.L. (1983): Control of proliferation of hepatocytes by two serum Hepatopoietins. Federation Proceedings 42:1023.

Miyazawa, K., Kitamura, A., Naka, D., and Kitamura, N. (1991): An alternatively processed mRNA generated from human hepatocyte growth factor gene. Eur. J. Biochem. 197:15-22.

Miyazawa, K., Tsubouchi, H., Naka, D., Takahashi, K., Okigaki, M., Arakaki, N., et al. (1989): Molecular cloning and sequence analysis of cDNA for human hepatocyte growth factor. Biochem. Biophys. Res. Commun. 163:967-973

Moolten, F.L., and Bucher, N.L.R. (1967): Regeneration of rat liver: Transfer of humoral agents by cross circulation. Science 158:272-274.

Nakamura, T., Nishizawa, T., Hagiya, M., Seki, T., Shimonishi, M., Sugimura, A., et al. (1989): Molecular cloning and expression of human hepatocyte growth factor. Nature 342:440-443.

Nakamura, T., Nawa, K., Ichihara, A., Kaise, N., and Nishino, T. (1987): Purification and subunit structure of hepatocyte growth factor from rat platelets. FEBS Letters 224:311-316.

Nakamura, T., Nawa, K., and Ichihara, A. (1984): Partial purification and characterization of hepatocyte growth factor from serum of hepatectomized rats. Biochem. Biophys. Res. Commun. 122:1450-1459.

Naldini, L., Vigna, E., Narsimhan, R.P., Gaudino, G., Zarnegar, R., Michalopoulos, G.K., et al. (1991): Hepatocyte growth factor (HGF) stimulates the tyrosine kinase activity of the receptor encoded by the proto-oncogene c-MET. Oncogene 1991; 6(4):501-4.

Noji, S., Tashiro, K., Koyama, E., Nohno, T., Ohyama, K., Taniguchi, S., et al. (1990): Expression of hepatocyte growth factor gene in endothelial and Kupffer cells of damaged rat livers, as revealed by in situ hybridization. Biochem. Biophys. Res. Commun. 173:42-47.

Okajima, A., Miyazawa, K., and Kitamura, N. (1990): Primary structure of rat hepatocyte growth factor and induction of its mRNA during liver regeneration following hepatic injury. Eur. J. Biochem. 193:375-81.

Rao, M.S., and Subbarao, V. (1986): DNA synthesis in exocrine and endocrine pancreas after partial hepatectomy in Syrian golden hamsters. Experientia 42:833-834.

Roesel, J., Rigsby, D., Bailey, A., Alvarez, R., Sanchez, J.D., Campbell, K., et al. (1989): Stimulation of protooncogene expression by partial hepatectomy is not tissue specific. Oncogene Research 5:129-136.

Rosen, E.M., Goldberg, I.D., Kacinski, B.M., Buckholz, T., and Vinter, D.W. (1989) Smooth muscle releases an epithelial cell scatter factor which binds to heparin. In Vitro Cell Dev. Biol. 1989;25:163-73.

Rubin, J.S., Chan, A.M., Bottaro, D.P., Burgess, W.H., Taylor,W.G., Chech, A.C., et al. (1991): A broad-spectrum human lung fibroblast-derived mitogen is a variant of hepatocyte growth factor. Proc. Natl. Acad Sci USA 88:415-419.

Russell, W.E., McGowan, J.A., and Bucher, N.L.R. (1984): Biological Properties of a Hepatocyte Growth Factor From Rat Platelets. Journal of Cellular Physiology 119:193-197.

Schirmacher, P., Geerts, A., Pietrangelo, A., Dienes, H.P., and Rogler, C.E. (1992): Hepatocyte Growth Factor/Hepatopoietin A is expressed in fat storing cells from rat liver but not myofibroblast-like cells derived from fat storing cells. Hepatology 15:5-11.

Seki, T., Hagiya, M., Shimonishi, M., Nakamura, T., and Shimizu S. (1991): Organization of the human hepatocyte growth factor-encoding gene. Gene 102:213-219.

Seki, T., Ihara, I., Sugimura, A., Shimmonishi, M., Nishizawa, T., Asami, O., et al. (1990): Isolation and expression of cDNA from different forms of Hepatocyte Growth Factor from human leucocyte. Biochem. Biophys. Res. Commun. 172:321-327.

Selden, C., Jones, M., Wade, D., and Hodgson, H. (1990): Hepatotropin mRNA expression in human foetal liver development and in liver regeneration. FEBS Lett 270:81-84.

Shimizu, I., Ichihara, A., and Nakamura, T. (1991): Hepatocyte growth factor in ascites from patients with cirrhosis. J Biochem (Tokyo) 109:14-18.

Stern, C.D., Ireland, G.W., Herrick, S.E., Gherardi, E., Gray, J., Perryman, M., et al. (1990): Epithelial scatter factor and development of the chick embryonic axis. Development 110:1271-1284.

Stoker, M., Gherardi, E., Perryman, M., and Gray, J. (1987): Scatter factor is a fibroblast-derived modulator of epithelial cell mobility. Nature 327(6119):239-42.

Strain, A.J., Ismail, T., Tsubouchi, H., Arakaki, N., Hishida, T., Kitamura, N., et al. (1991): Native and recombinant human hepatocyte growth factors are highly potent promoters of DNA synthesis in both human and rat hepatocytes. J. Clin. Invest. 87:1853-1857.

Tashiro, K., Hagiya, M., Nishizawa, T., Seki, T., Shimonishi, M., Shimizu, S., et al. (1990): Deduced primary structure of rat hepatocyte growth factor and expression of the mRNA in rat tissues. Proc. Natl. Acad. Sci. USA 87:3200-3204.

Tomiya, T., Nagoshi, S., and Fujiwara, K. (1992): Significance of serum human Hepatocyte Growth Factor levels in patients with hepatic failure. Hepatology 15:1-4.

Tsubouchi, H., Hirono, S., Gohda, E., Nakayama, H., Takahashi, K., Sakiyama, O., et al. (1991): Human hepatocyte growth factor in blood of patients with fulminant hepatic failure. I. Clinical aspects. Dig. Dis. Sci. 36:780-784.

Tsubouchi, H., Niitani, Y., Hirono, S., Nakayama, H., Gohda, E., et al. (1991): Levels of the human hepatocyte growth factor in serum of patients with various liver diseases determined by an enzyme-linked immunosorbent assay. Hepatology 13:1-5.

Weidner, M., Arakaki, N., Hartmann, G., Vandekerckhove, J., Weingart, S., Rieder, H, et al. (1991): Evidence for the identity of human scatter factor and human hepatocyte growth factor. Proc. Natl. Acad. Sci. (USA) 88:7001-7005.

Wolf, H.K., Zarnegar, R., and Michalopoulos, G.K. (1991): Localization of Hepatocyte Growth Factor in human and rat tissues: An immunohistochemical study. Hepatology 14:488-494.

Wolf, H., Zarnegar, R., Oliver, L., and Michalopoulos, G.K. (1991): Hepatocyte Growth Factor (HGF) in human placenta and trophoblastic disease. Amer. J. Path., 138:1035-1043.

Yoshiyama, Y., Arakaki, N., Naka, D., Takahashi, K., Hirono, S., Kondo, J., et al. (1991): Identification of the N-terminal residue of the heavy chain of both native and recombinant human hepatocyte growth factor. Biochem. Biophys. Res. Commun. 175:660-667.

Zarnegar, R., DeFrances, M.C., Kost, D.P., Lindroos, P., and Michalopoulos, G.K. (1991): Expression of hepatocyte growth factor mRNA in regenerating rat liver after partial hepatectomy. Biochem. Biophys. Res. Commun. 177:559-565.

Zarnegar, R., DeFrances, M., and Michalopoulos, G.K. Localization of the human HGF gene on chromosome 7. Genomics, In Press.

Zarnegar, R., DeFrances, M.C., Oliver, L., and Michalopoulos, G. (1990): Identification and partial characterization of receptor binding sites for HGF on rat hepatocytes. Biochem. Biophys. Res. Commun. 173:1179-1185.

Zarnegar, R., and Michalopoulos, G. (1989): Purification and Biological Characterization of Human Hepatopoietin A, a Polypeptide Growth Factor for Hepatocytes. Cancer Research 49:3314-3320.

Zarnegar, R., Muga, S., Enghild, J., and Michalopoulos, G. (1989): NH2-terminal amino acid sequence of rabbit hepatopoietin A, a heparin-binding polypeptide growth factor for hepatocytes. Biochem. Biophys. Res. Commun., 163:1370-1376.

Zarnegar, R., Muga, S., Rahija, R., and Michalopoulos, G.K. (1990): Tissue distribution of HPTA, a heparin-binding polypeptide growth factor for hepatocytes. Proc. Nat. Acad. Sci. (USA) 87:1252-1256.

Liver Regeneration. Eds D. Bernuau, G. Feldmann. John Libbey Eurotext, Paris © 1992, pp. 103-115.

Insulin-like growth factor II (IGF-II) in human primary liver cancer : a progression factor and/or a marker of liver cell differentiation

C. Bréchot, F. Zindy, E. Cariani, E. Lamas, C. Lasserre

INSERM U.75, CHU Necker, 156 rue de Vaugirard, 75742 Paris Cedex 15.
Unité d'Hépatologie, Hôpital Laennec, 42 rue de Sèvres, 75007 Paris, France

Introduction

IGF-II is a polypeptide structurally homologous to insulin, insulin-like growth factor I and relaxin. The role of IGF-II is unknown although is it synthetized in several fetal tissues and might stimulate fetal growth (1). The genetic organization and transcriptional regulation of IGF-II gene is complex and includes alternative splicing of different 5' untranslated exons (2-7). The pattern of IGF-II transcripts in the liver is both tissue specific and developmental stage dependent ; indeed three major IGF-II mRNAs (6,5.3, and 4.8-5 kilobases in size) have been identified which are generated from distinct promoters and, possibly, by differential splicing (Fig.1) (7-11). The activation of a first promoter would generate in normal adult liver a 5.3-kilobase mRNA, including the 3 coding exons and the 5'-untranslated regions designated as non coding exons 1,2, and 3. Alternatively, the activation of a second promoter would generate in fetal liver a 6-kilobase mRNA, including the 3 coding exons and the 5'-untranslated region designated as non coding exon 4. In addition, the existence of a third and a fourth promoter has been established, which would be located in a distinct 5'-untranslated DNA sequence (19) ; this third promoter would generate a 4.8-5-kilobase transcript identified in Wilms' tumor, fetal liver, and placenta. The importance of IGF-II as a mitogen as well as the role of IGF-II receptor are still debated. The IGF-II receptor has been recently cloned and characterized ; its structure differs from that of IGF-I and insulin receptor genes. In fact, the IGF-II receptor is identical to the cation-independent mannose 6-phosphate (CIM6P) receptor, involved in the targeting of lysosomal enzymes to lysosomes.
High levels of IGF-II mRNA were found in several human and rodent fetal tissues (including liver, kidney, and striated muscle) whereas, in the adult, the same tissues showed less abundant IGF-II mRNA expression. An elevation od IGF-II transcripts was shown in some embryonic tumors, such as nephroblastoma (Wilms' tumor) and rhabdomyosarcoma which originate from tissues normally expressing high levels of IGF-II mRNA during the fetal life. Deletions in the short arm of chromosome 11, where IGF-II gene is located (band 11p15),

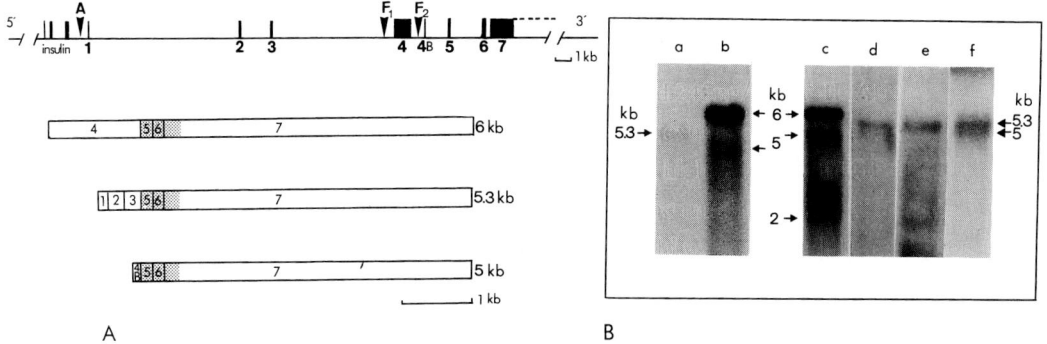

Figure 1 : **Genetic organization of the IGF-II gene.**
A shows the structure of 3 RNAs generated from the adult (A) and the 2 fetal (F1 and F2) promoters. A fourth promoter, recently described (19), is not indicated in this figure.
B shows representative example of fetal and adult IGF-II RNA profiles.

have recently been identified as a potentially common tumorigenic mechanism in different embryonic tumors, including nephroblastoma, rhabdomyosarcoma, and hepatoblastoma. The overexpression of IGF-II mRNA observed in Wilms' tumor might be related to these deletions. Some studies indicate the possibility of a modified IGF-II expression in human primary liver tumors. Indeed, rearrangements of chromosome 11 have been described in a human hepatocellular carcinoma, as well as in hepatoblastoma. Although no data are presently available on human primary liver tumors, the hepatoblastoma cell line Hep-G2 exhibits increased levels of IGF-II mRNA, as well as a fetal pattern of transcripts. An elevation of IGF-II mRNA was also recently shown in woodchucks primary liver tumors (6,8). This led to the hypothesis that IGF-II may play a role in the deregulation of growth control in hepatocytes upon their transformation into tumorous cells.

Aims of the study

The aims of our investigations were therefore :
1) to analyze the IGF-II expression in vivo, both at the mRNA and protein levels, in human primary liver cancer, benign liver tumors and cirrhotic liver.
2) To identify the liver cell types involved in IGF-II synthesis.
3) To evaluate the influence of liver cell differenciation on IGF-II expression profil.

Methods

IGF-II RNA was analyzed with dot-blot and Northern blots using an IGF-II cDNA derived from human fetal liver and oligonucleotide probes corresponding to the non coding exons 4 and 4B.
- IGF-II protein was tested in serum and liver using a radio immuno assay based on IGF-II binding proteins (9).
- The localisation of the IGF-II mRNAs and proteins was tested through 2 complementary approaches :
* in situ hybridization
* isolation and primary culture of rat hepatocytes and non parenchymal liver cells.

Results

1) IGF-II mRNA and protein liver tumors and cirrhosis (12)

1.1 Hybridization with IGF-II cDNA showed a significant increase of IGF-II mRNA in nine of the 40 (22%) liver cancer samples (Fig 2 and Table 1)
This increase of IGF-II mRNA was generally only observed in the tumorous area, although non tumorous liver also showed increased IGF-II mRNA in three cases. All of the non tumorous areas which showed IGF-II overexpression were cirrhotic, whereas histologically normal non tumorous liver did not show any evidence of increased IGF-II mRNA. By contrast with liver cancers, IGF-II mRNA levels in bening tumors and cirrhosis were comparable to those observed in normal adult liver.
Hybridization with a fetal liver IGF-II cDNA probe showed distinct patterns according to the liver samples analyzed. The simultaneous detection of 6- and 5-kilobase fetal mRNAs was mainly observed in primary liver cancers, including all the samples with an increase in IGF-II mRNA. By contrast, this pattern was shown in only two benign liver tumors (one of these being associated with a hepatocellular carcinoma) and in none of the cirrhosis without associated cancer. The presence of the 5.3-kilobase adult transcript was mainly identified in benign liver tumors and cirrhosis without associated cancer, it was also present in some liver cancer samples in tumorous and non tumorous areas. The presence of both adult 5.3- and fetal 5-kilobase transcripts was only identified in some benign liver tumors and liver cirrhosis. These results were confirmed by hybridizing the same filters with oligonucleotide probes specific for non coding exons 4 and 4B.

1.2 IGF-II protein content was tested by a protein-binding assay (9) in a series of eleven liver cancer samples and compared with IGF-II mRNA status (13) (Table 2).

In the reference normal adult liver samples IGF-II protein content ranged from 17-73ng:g (mean 41.3 ± 18.7). The one fetal liver sample tested contained 245ng/g IGF-II. All the examined tumorous areas and eight of the non-tumorous areas exhibited an elevation of IGF-II protein as compared to normal adult liver. Furthermore, the highest levels of IGF-II (450-1280ng/g, 10-30-fold vs. normal adult liver) were detected in the tumorous areas with the largest increases in the expression of IGF-II mRNA (90-150-fold vs. normal adult liver). Ten of the eleven primary liver cancer samples contained more IGF-II protein in tumorous than non-tumorous areas, although the difference varied (the ratios for tumorous to non-tumorous IGF-II ranged from 1.2-6.5). Therefore this demonstrates an increased IGF-II expression both at the mRNA and protein level in the tumors. It should be noted however that there was not a strict correlation between IGF-II protein and mRNA levels.

This result is consistent with observations made in Wilms' tumor, where IGF-II mRNA levels were 30-times higher than in normal kidney but without a corresponding increase in the amount of IGF-II. On the other hand, in pheochromocytoma, a 4-fold rise in IGF-II mRNA content was accompanied by a 100-fold rise in the amount of IGF-II.

Interestingly, the simultaneous determination of IGF-I mRNA and protein content in the liver cancer samples did not show significant increases as compared to normal liver.

2) Localisation of liver cell types expressing IGF-II in tumors and normal liver (14, 15, 16).

2.1 In situ hybridization (14)

In normal human liver sections, IGF-II mRNAs were detected exclusively in the hepatocytes. All hepatocytes were labeled and no zonal variation in the intensity of labeling within the hepatic lobules was observed. The distribution of silver grains was similar to that obtained with an albumin probe. However, the number of silver grains was very low wtih the IGF-II probe. In our experimental conditions no signal was observed in the sinusoidal cells.

In liver sections from three patients with liver cancer, two of them with a well differentiated hepatocarcinoma, the labeling was homogeneously observed in most tranformed hepatocytes in the tumoral tissue. The intensity of signal was estimated to be 2 to 5 times stronger than in normal liver tissue, equivalent to that found with the albumin probe.

In contrast, in sections from non tumoral tissue at distance from the tumor, a very weak signal was observed in all hepatocytes. However, an intense labeling was detected in some regenerative nodules. The cells labeled in theses nodules had a morphologic appearance consistent with that previously described for dysplastic hepatocytes. Using IGF-II sense probe, no signal was detected in normal liver tissue.

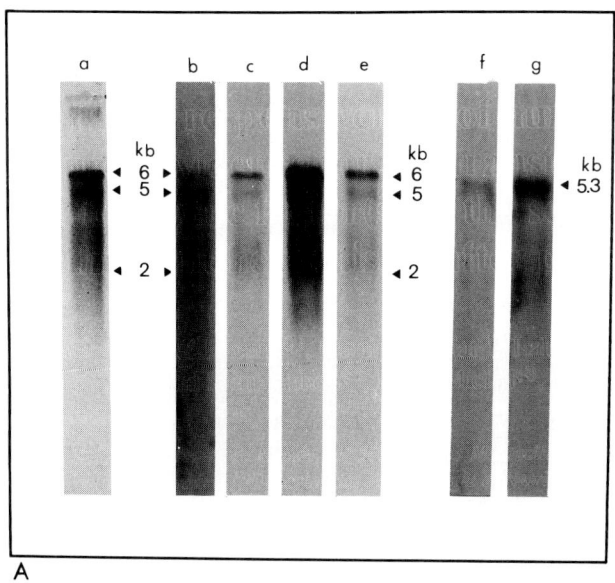

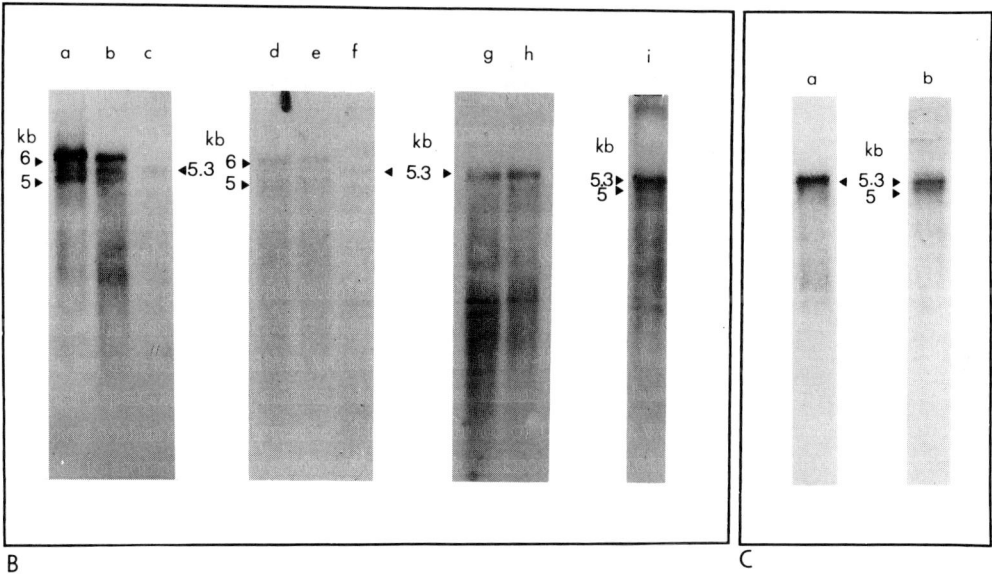

Figure 2 : **Northern blot analysis of RNA extracted from tumorous and non tumorous livers from patients with HCC, and probed with an IGF-II cDNA.**
The 6, 5kb and 2kb RNA molecules are fetal IGF-II transcripts while the 5.3kb RNA is an adult IGF-II RNA. Lans a-e show samples with reexpression of a fetal IGF-II pattern while the lanes f and g show an adult IGF-II RNA profile.

TABLE 1
IGF-II mRNA pattern in primary liver cancers, benign tumors and liver cirrhosis

	IGF-II mRNA pattern		5.3-kilobase (Adult)
	6-kilobase (Fetal) 5-kilobase (Fetal)	5.3-kilobase (Adult) 5-kilobase (Fetal)	
Primary liver cancers			
Tumorous tissue (19)	14*	0	5
Non Tumorous tissue (17)	7†	0	10
Benign liver cancers			
Tumorous tissue (12)	2	1	9
Non Tumorous tissue (11)	0	1	10
Liver cirrhosis (8)	0	3	5

* 9/14 had increased IGF-II mRNA level.
† All histological cirrhosis. 3/17 had increased IGF-II mRNA levels. One of these samples showed also a 5.3-kilobase transcript.

IGF-II protein was detected in the cytoplasm of hepatocytes in both tumoral and peritumoral liver tissues including some dysplastic hepatocytes. The specificity of the staining was supported by its extinction after adsorption with human recombinant IGF-II.

2.2 <u>Expression of IGF-II in isolated hepatocytes and non parenchymal rat liver cells</u> (15, 16).

2.2.1. <u>Expression of IGF-II mRNA in vivo : freshly isolated rat hepatocytes during development and in fetal and adult rat liver tissues</u>. IGF-II mRNA was detectable in the freshly isolated hepatocytes taken from fetal, newborn and adult rat liver. Rat hepatocytes isolated between the seventeenth day of gestation and the seventeenth day after birth expressed the five RNA transcripts for IGF-II ; this pattern of expression corresponds to that previously found in fetal liver tissue (4.6, 3.6, 2.2, 1.6 and 1.2kb). The amount of IGF-II RNA decreases dramatically after the seventeenth day after birth. As of the twenty-first day after birth, isolated hepatocytes showed a change in the pattern of expression for IGF-II RNAs.

Table 2

IGF-II Content of Liver and Serum Samples

A : primary liver cancer with a fetal IGF-II transcript pattern, showing IGF-II mRNA overexpression in tumorous and/or non tumorous areas. B : primary liver cancer expressing a fetal IGF-II transcript pattern, without overexpression. C : primary liver cancer with an adult liver IGF-II transcript pattern. T : tumorous area. NT : non tumorous area.

* : samples overexpressing IGF-II mRNA.
° : samples displaying a fetal IGF-II mRNA pattern without overexpression.

		LIVER IGF-II (ng/g)			Serum IGF-II (ng/ml)
		T	NT	T/NT	normal range 1073-1216
Group A	**Primary Liver Cancers**				
	D.	114 *	189 *	0.6	263
	K.	450 *	100	4.5	530
	B.	850 *	190	4.5	415
	N.	142 *	58	2.4	-----
	F.	144 °	121 *	1.2	1342
	Fi.	1280 *	197 °	6.5	319
Group B	O.	341 °	195	1.7	-----
	G.	285 °	128 °	2.2	320
	C.	200 °	132	1.5	533
Group C	Cl.	81	70	1.1	-----
	L.	163	85	1.9	-----
	Adult Liver				
	Y		34)		
	505		17)		
	510		34)	(mean 41.3 ± 18.7)	
	516		48)		
	503		73)		
	504		42)		
	Fetal Liver		245		

Two mRNA species (1.6 and 1.2kb) characteristic of adult liver tissues were observed in hepatocytes isolated from 2-mo-old rats. The accumulation of IGF-II RNA in hepatocytes isolated from either 21-day-old rats or adults was similar to that observed in vivo (adult liver tissue).

2.2.2. Expression of IGF-II gene in vitro : primary culture of adult rat hepatocytes.

IGF-II mRNA was detectable in several independent experiments throughout the primary culture of adult hepatocytes (from the first to the eight day). Two mRNA species, 1.6 and 1.2kb, encoding IGF-II, were observed in these cells. This pattern of expression of IGF-II is the same as that found in normal adult liver. IGF-II protein was detectable in the hepatocyte culture medium (Fig 3).

IGF-II, IGF-I and insulin receptor mRNAs were also shown in the adult rat hepatocytes in culture.

In addition to IGF-II mRNA, IGF-II protein synthesis and secretion by hepatocytes was also evidenced. Thus, adult rat hepatocytes conserve a correct tissue-specific expression in culture, and the expression of these genes does not depend on cell interactions normally present in the intact liver.

2.2.3. Expression of IGF-II in sinusoidal cells (16)

IGF-II mRNA was detectable in the different non parenchymal liver cells isolated from 10-, 18- and 60-day- old male Wistar rats. In Kupffer and endothelial cells from 10-day-old rats, the IGF-II transcripts were identical (4.6,6.3,2.2,1.6,1.2kb) to fetal rat hepatocytes. By 18 days, the amount of IGF-II mRNAs was markedly reduced and ony the 3.6, 1.6 and 1.2kb transcripts were shown. At 60 days, only two transcripts were detected (1.6 and 1.2kb). This pattern was identical to the pattern in adult rat hepatocytes.

In contrast, in fat-storing cells only the 3.6, 1.6 and 1.2kb IGF-II mRNAs were detected in 10-day-old animals. In addition, only the 1.6 and 1.2kb mRNA molecules (i.e., the adult IGF-II mRNA profile) were demonstrated in 18- and 60-day-old rats.

The three receptor mRNA species (IGF-I, IGF-II and insulin) were expressed in all cell types. This study demonstrates that IGF-II expression occurs in the three different sinusoidal liver cell types isolated through centrifugal elutrition, in accordance with previous results (11).

3. IGF-II expression according to the liver cell differenciation status (17-18).

3.1. IGF-II and HBV transcripts in liver cancer (17)

HBV markers (especially HBcAg, associated with viral replication) are rarely found in

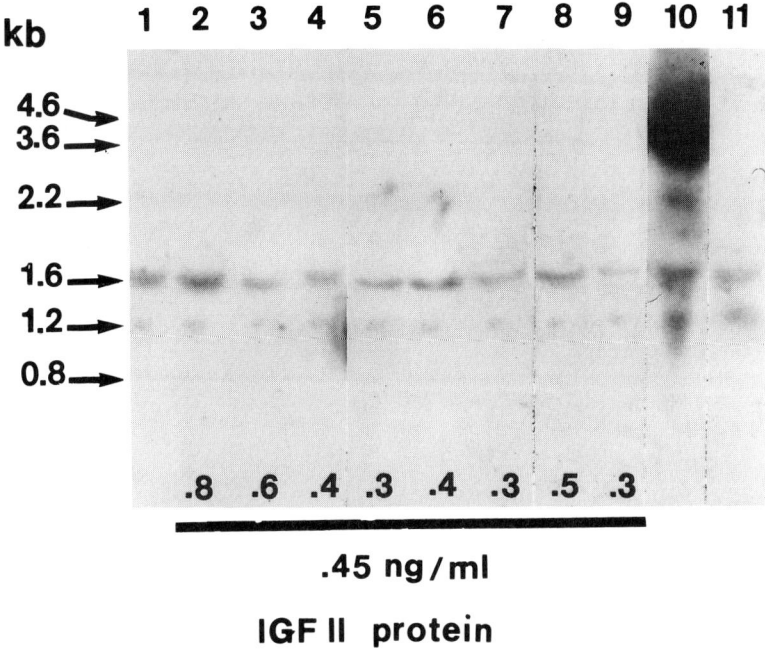

Figure 3 : **Expression of IGF-II RNA and protein in primary culture of rat hepatocytes.**
Two adult IGF-II RNAs (1.6 and 1.2kb) are detected throughout the culture. Secretion of IGF-II protein in the medium is also evidenced.

neoplastic cells, whereas they can be detected in nontumorous liver surrounding liver cancer. This observation supports the hypothesis that HBV replication becomes less active during the process of hepatocarcinogenesis and is consistent with the fact that HBV RNA is mostly observed in nonneoplastic liver surrounding liver cancer. Recent evidence in woodchuck HCC showed a relationship between the dgree of HCC differentiation and the expression of IGF-II and woodchuk hepatitis virus (WHV) transcripts (6,8). HCCs with low IGF-II mRNA and high WHV RNA levels were generally highly differentiated, whereas tumors with IGF-II mRNA and low WHV RNA levels were more anaplastic.

To analyze the possible relevance of IGF-II mRNA as a marker of hepatocyte differentiation and transformation, we compared IGF-II mRNA pattern and AFP mRNA expression in the same tumorous and nontumorous liver samples from 16 human primary liver cancers (mostly highly differentiated HCCs). HBV RNA was also analyzed in seven liver cancers from HBV chronic caarriers.

TABLE 3
Comparative analysis of AFP mRNA and fetal IGFII mRNA expression in primary liver cancer
(16 tumorous and 17 nontumorous areas)

Primary liver cancers		AFP mRNA	IGFII mRNA fetal patern
T (16)	4	+	+
	5	−	+
	7	−	−
NT (17)	1	+	+
	6	−	+
	10	−	−

Histological examination of nontumorous liver samples showed that 12 tumors were surrounded by cirrhotic tissue and four by histologically normal liver.

Eleven of the liver cancers in this series did not display AFP mRNA expression in the tumorous or nontumorous areas. Most of these tumors (10 out of 11) were highly differentiated, and one was moderately differentiated. IGF-II mRNA was increased in two tumorous and one nontumorous sample not expressing AFP mRNA. Furthermore, Northern blot analysis showed that fetal IGF-II transcripts were expressed in these samples and in three additional tumorous tissues and four nontumorous cirrhotic areas not showing AFP or increased IGF-II mRNA expression. Therefore fetal IGF-II transcripts were more frequently observed than AFP mRNA both in highly differentiated human liver cancers and the surrounding cirrhotic tissues (Table 3).

Seven of the liver cancer patients included in this series were HBV chrnoic carriers. HBV RNA was analyzed both in tumorous and nontumorous tissues from these patients.

IGF-II mRNA pattern was analyzed in all the above samples. Two tumors, in which HBV transcripts were not detectable, showed a fetal pattern of IGF-II transcripts associated with increased IGF-II mRNA expression. The remaining five paired tumorous-nontumorous samples from chronic HBV carriers had low IGF-II mRNA levels associated, when detectable, with an adult IGF-II transcript of 5.3kb.

3.2 IGF-II expression during hepatocarcinogenes in transgenic mice (18)

The injection into mouse eggs of a transgene containing the early region of SV40 under the control of the human antithrombin III (ATIII) regulatory sequences leads to the developement of hepatocellular carcinomas (HCCs) around the age of 7 months in heterozygous animals (11). The development of HCC is preceded by the appearance of nuclear and cellular alterations (anisocytosis, anisocaryosis) at 2 months, the development of clear cell nodules at 3 months and of liver adenomas at 6 months. In this model we examined, at different steps of liver cell transformation, the steady-state level of IGF-II mRNA and of other differentiation-related mRNAs : alphafetoprotein (AFP) ; ornithine transcarbamylase (OTC), which is specifically expressed in liver and intestine ; and SV40 early region transgene which, being under the control of ATIII regulatory sequences, is specifically expressed in liver tissue.

Liver samples from heterozygous (3 to 8 months) and homozygous (6 months) transgenics were studied. Macroscopic nodules were isolated and analyzed separately from surrounding liver tissue.

With regard to RNA isolated from total liver, IGF-II cDNA probe only hybridized to samples from an 8-month heterozygous and a 6-month homozygous. Both these tissues consisted of histologically differentiated HCCs.

When isolated liver nodules were analyzed, IGF-II mRNA was detected in a cancerous nodule from the 8-month heterozygous and in one of three cancerous nodules from the 6-month homozygous. On the contrary, IGF-II mRNA was not detected in other two nodules from the same animal, both differentiated HCCs. In addition, two macroscopic nodules isolated from a 3-month heterozygous transgenic showed a strong expression of IGF-II mRNA, which was not detectable in surrounding liver. The two nodules mainly contained clear cells, and did not show any histological character of malignant transformation.

In this model therefore, a fetal pattern of IGF-II can be reexpressed in cells which do not show a complete transformed phenotype.

Conclusions

The pattern of IGF-II expression during the different steps of liver cell transfomration suggests 2, non exclusive, hypothesis :

1) IGF-II can be viewed as a marker of liver cell differenciation, its fetal profil being reexpressed during liver carcinogenesis. In this view, our results indicate that IGF-II might be an early marker of malignant cell proliferation.

2) IGF-II has been shown to be, at least in some experimental model, to be a mitogenic factors. However this has not been demonstrated for hepatocytes in vitro. It is therefore plausible that IGF-II is acting during progression of the liver carcinogenesis after initiation of the tumor development by other factors.

Références

1. Froesch, E.R., Schmid, C., Schwander, J., and Zapf, J. Actions of insulin like growth factors. Ann. Rev. Physiol., 47 : 443-467, 1985.

2. de Pagter-Holthuizen, P., Van Schaik, F., M. A., Verduijn, G. M., Van Ommen, G.J.B., Bouma, B.N., Jansen, M., and Sussenbach, J.S. Organization of the human genes for insulin-like growth factors I and II variants. FEBS Lett., 179 : 243-246, 1985.

3. Scott, J., Cowell, J., Robertson, M.E., Priestley, L.M., Wadey, R., Hopkins, B., Pritchard, J., Bell, G.I., Rall, L.B., Graham, C.F., and Knott, T.J. Insulin-like growth factor-II gene expression in Wilms' tumor and embryonic tissues. Nature (Lond), 317 : 260-262, 1985.

4. Tricoli, J.V., Rall; L.B., Scott, J., Bell, G.I., and Showd, T.B. Localization of insulin-like growth factor genes to human chromosomes 11 and 12. Nature (Lond), 310 : 784-786, 1984.

5. Rogler, C.E., Sherman, M., Su, C.Y., Shafritz, D.A., Summers, J., Shows, T.B., Henderson, A. and Kew, M. Deletion in chromosome 11p associated with a hepatitis B integration site in hepatocellular carcinoma. Science (Wash. DDC), 230 : 319-322, 1985.

6. Rogler, C.E., Hino, O., and Su, C.Y. Molecular aspects of persistent woodchuck hepatitis virus and hepatitis B virus infection and hepatocellular carcinoma. Hepatology, 7 : 74S-78S, 1987.

7. Brice, L.A, Cheetham, E.J., Boltonh, H.V., Hill, W.C.N., Schofield P. Temporal changes in the expression of the insulin-like growth factor II gene associated with tissue maturation in the human fetus. Development 106 : 543, 1989.

8. Xi-Xian F., Chun Yeh S., Young L., Ray, H., Biempica, L., Snydem, Roger, Ch. Insulin-like growth factor II expression and oval cell proliferation associated with hepatocarcinogenesis in wood chuck hepatitis virus carries. J. Virol. 3422, 1988.

9. Binoux, M., Lasserre, C., Gourmelon, M. Specific assay for insulin-like growth factor (IGF) II using the IGF binding proteins extracted from human cerebrospinal fluid. J. Clin. Endocrinol. Metab. 1986, 63 : 1151-1155.

10. Han, V.K.M., D'Ercole, A.J., Lund, P.K. Cellular localization of somatomedin (insulin-like growth factor) messenger RNA in the human fetus. Science 236 : 193, 1987.

11. Dubois, N., Bennoun, M.M., Allemand, I. et al. Time-course development of differentiated hepatocarcinoma and lung metastasis in transgenic mice. J. Hepatol. 13 : 227-39, 1991.

12. Cariani, E., Lasserre, C., Seurin, D., Hamelin, B., Kemeny, F., Franco, D., Czech, MP., Ullrich, A., Bréchot, C. Differential expression of insulin like-growth factor II mRNA in human primary liver cancers, benign liver tumors, and liver cirrhosis.Cancer research 48, 6844-6849.

13. Cariani, E., Seurin, D., Lasserre, C., Franco, D., Binoux, M., Bréchot, C. Expression of insulin-like growth factor II (IGF-II) in human primary liver cancer : mRNA and protein analysis. J. Hepatol. 1990, 11 : 226-231.

14. Lamas, E., Le Bail, B., Housset, C., Boucher, O., Bréchot C. Localization of insulin like growth factor II and hepatitis B virus mRNAs and proteins in human hepatocellular carcinomas. Laboratory investigation 64 : 98-104.

15. Lamas, E., Zindy, F., Seurin, D., Guguen-Guillouzo, C., Bréchot, C. Expression of insulin-like growth factor II and receptors for insulin-like growth factor II, insulin -like growth factor I and insulin in isolated and cultured rat hepatocytes. Hepatology, 13 : 936-940.

16. Zindy, F., Lamas, E. Schmidt, S., Kirn, A., Bréchot, C. Expression of insulin-like growth factor II (IGF-II) and IGF-II, IGF-I and insulin receptors mRNAs in isolated non parenchymal rat liver cells. J. Hepatol.1992 ; 14 : 30-34

17. Cariani, E., Lasserre, C., Kemeny, F., Franco, D., Bréchot, C. Expression of insulin-like growth factor II, alpha-fetoprotein and hepatitis B virus transcripts in human primary liver cancer. Hepatology 13, 644-649.

18. Cariani, E., Dubois, N., Lasserre, C., Briand, P., Bréchot, C. Insulin-like growth factor II (IGF-II) mRNA expression during hepatocarcinogenesis in transgenic mice. Journal of Hepatology, 1991 ; 13 : 220-226.

19. Van Dijk, MA., Van Shaik, F.F.A., Bootsma, H.J., Holthuizen, P. and Sussenbach, J.S. Initial characterisation of the human insulin-like growth factor II gene. Mol. and cellular endocrinology. 1991, 81 : 81-94.

Alpha-fetoprotein and hepatocyte proliferation

D. Bernuau, I. Tournier, J.Y. Scoazec, G. Feldmann

Laboratoire de Biologie Cellulaire INSERM U.327, Faculté de Médecine Xavier Bichat, Paris, France

The alpha-fetoprotein (AFP) gene is a characteristic example of a developmentally regulated gene. It is expressed at high levels in the liver and the yolk sac during the fetal life and its expression is turned off after birth, to reach almost undetectable levels during normal adult life (Abelev, 1971). Inhibition of AFP gene expression in differentiated hepatocytes appears to be reversible. Indeed, AFP production resumes temporarily during liver regeneration and hepatocyte proliferation *in vitro* (Abelev,1971; Petropoulos *et al.*,1983). Moreover, hepatocyte transformation is frequently concomitant with a strong activation of the gene (Abelev,1971). The mechanisms of AFP gene regulation during normal liver development, liver regeneration and carcinogenesis are still uncompletely understood, although it is now clear that such regulation is mainly at the transcriptional level. In this report we present data based on analysis of AFP gene expression at the cellular level which support a link between hepatocyte replication and activation of the AFP gene.

I. Correlation between AFP expression and hepatocyte replication during liver development :

During embryonic development, expression of the AFP gene becomes first detectable in 9-day mouse embryo, before the start of liver morphogenesis (Schmid & Schulz,1990) and the gene is abundantly expressed throughout subsequent liver development. Albumin mRNA appear one day later, when cord formation starts (Shiojiri *et al.*,1991). Hematopoetic cells which invade the liver during days 10 and 11 of gestation do not express the AFP gene at any stage. The proliferation rate of fetal hepatocytes is very high. It is now well demonstrated that all fetal hepatocytes, and not a fraction of them, express the AFP gene concomitantly with the albumin gene (Poliard *et al.*,1986; Schmid & Schultz,1990; Shiojiri *et al.*,1991). After birth, transcription of the AFP gene declines rapidly, with a fall in the liver concentration of AFP mRNA, and a decrease in the amount of AFP transcript per cell, on in situ hybridization (Poliard *et al.*,1986). Such a decline is concomitant with a decrease of the proliferative activity of neonatal hepatocytes.

During the first post-natal week, a zonal lobular heterogeneity in the level of AFP gene expression becomes evident, with a higher number of gene product (mRNA and protein) in perivenous than in periportal hepatocytes. This heterogeneity persists until the fourth week, when AFP mRNA sequences and protein are barely detectable (Poliard *et al.*,1986). A link between the proliferative capacity of neonatal hepatocytes and the higher level of expression of the AFP gene in the perivenous hepatocytes would imply a higher proliferative capacity of hepatocytes around the central vein during the post-natal period. The results of *in vivo* radioactive thymidine incorporation indicate, on the contrary, that the decline of the proliferative activity of neonatal hepatocytes after birth occurs first in perivenous hepatocytes (Le Bouton,1974). These data suggest that the perinatal lobular heterogeneity of AFP expression is related to repression of gene transcription which operates specifically at this period. A glucocorticoid responsive element on the AFP gene promoter has been identified as a negative regulatory factor (Nakabayashi et al.,1989; Poliard et al.,1990)). This element might be implicated in the post-natal repression of AFP transcription which has been shown to be influenced by glucocorticoids (Bélanger et al.,1981). The faster decrease of AFP mRNA in periportal neonatal hepatocytes could be related to differences in glucocorticoid concentrations or to a higher sensitivity of periportal hepatocytes than perivenous hepatocytes to these hormones. During liver maturation, there is a shift in the size of AFP mRNA. While fetal liver expresses a major 2.1 kb transcript, smaller variants of 1.4 and 1.0 kb are found in the adult liver (Wan & Chou,1989).

In the adult liver, the proliferation rate of hepatocytes is very low. AFP protein becomes undetectable by immunocytochemistry. Using a probe which detects predominantly the adult forms of AFP mRNA (1.4 and 1.0 kb transcripts), low level of expression of these mRNA were found in all adult hepatocytes, without any lobular zonation (Poliard et al.,1986). Lemire et al. have recently shown that the fetal 2.1 kb transcript is also expressed at very low level in the normal adult liver by some ductular cells, which have been hypothetically referred to as facultative stem cells, and by a few randomly distributed mature hepatocytes (Lemire & Fausto,1991).

II. AFP activation and proliferation of adult hepatocytes *in vivo* :

A) In rodents :
Liver regeneration is a demonstrative situation illustrating the relationship between hepatocyte proliferation and AFP gene reexpression by adult differentiated hepatocytes. AFP plasma levels increase after surgical or chemical partial hepatectomy in the rat. In young adult rats or mice, surgical removal of two-thirds of the liver mass elicits a dramatic proliferative response of the remaining hepatocytes leading to restoration of the liver mass within a few weeks. All adult hepatocytes participate to this regenerative response. Similarly, reactivation of the AFP gene at the mRNA level is detected by *in situ* hybridization in all hepatocytes of the remaining lobes, 48 h after partial hepatectomy (Bernuau et al.,1988). Interestingly, there is a striking correlation between the kinetics of hepatocyte proliferation and AFP gene activation. The proliferative response of hepatocytes begins in the periportal zones, and progresses in waves towards the central veins (Grisham,1962). Nuclear accumulation of AFP mRNA in the same way is first detected in periportal hepatocytes as soon as 2 h post-hepatectomy, that is during the early pre-replicative phase, suggesting that activation of AFP gene transcription is parallel to very early replicative events. Cytoplasmic accumulation of AFP mRNA is not detectable before 48 h , that is at a time when most hepatocytes have completed at least one round of cell division. These data suggest that nuclear AFP mRNA transport and translation is restricted to a post-S or post-mitotic phase of the cell cycle. The level of activation of AFP synthesis per cell remains relatively weak, since almost no hepatocytes stain for the protein after partial hepatectomy in the adult rat (Bernuau et al.,1988).

Acute chemical intoxication represents another model for the study of liver regeneration. In this situation, hepatocyte proliferation is preceeded by the occurence of liver cell necrosis, whose importance and lobular localization varies from one model to another. Acute intoxication with carbon tetrachloride induces within 48 h necrosis of the perivenous zones of the liver lobule, resulting in a one-third to two-thirds chemical hepatectomy. Proliferation of the majority of the remaining hepatocytes is induced in a relatively well synchronized manner, with a peak of mitotic activity by 48 h and 72 h. AFP gene transcription is activated as soon as 24 h after intoxication (Panduro et al.,1986), therefore again in the pre-replicative phase, while cytoplasmic AFP mRNA accumulation is observed within all hepatocytes at 48 and 72 h (Tournier et al.,1988). As for partial hepatectomy, therefore, AFP gene activation appears correlated with the entry of adult hepatocytes into the proliferative cycle.

After acute D-galactosamine intoxication, necrosis is primarily to hepatocytes but, although all cell types proliferate, hepatocyte DNA synthesis is weak , probably due to the fact that D-galactosamine metabolites impair hepatocyte RNA synthesis. As in other situations where hepatocyte replication is impaired, oval cells (which have the properties of progenitor cells) and bile duct cells proliferate. In this model, AFP gene activation is not detected in hepatocytes, but in the proliferated oval cells and in proliferated bile duct cells and some small hepatocytes derived from the oval cells (Tournier et al.,1988). In all these cell types, AFP mRNA are expressed as fetal type transcripts of full size (2.1 kb) (Lemire et al.,1991).

The development of a turpentine-induced acute inflammatory reaction in the adult rat is accompanied by an increase in the steady-state level of the nuclear oncogenes c-fos and c-myc mRNA, with a concomitant increase of AFP adult mRNA transcripts (1.7 and 1.0 kb).(D. Bernuau, submitted). Interestingly, in this situation neither stimulation of the incorporation of ^{3}-H thymidine in hepatocytes nor mitoses are observed. Thus, AFP activation in adult hepatocytes is not necessarily coupled with DNA synthesis and mitosis.

B) **In man :**
A relationship between hepatocyte proliferation and AFP gene activation appears less obvious than in animals. There is no detectable rise of AFP serum level after partial hepatectomy in man, whereas liver regeneration apparently proceeds normally (Alpert & Feller,1978). Several reasons could explain these observations. Strain and age-related differences in the level of AFP reactivation have been demonstrated during liver regeneration. For example, AFP activation is greater in mice than in rats, and in young animals compared to older animals. The majority of the patients studied were over the age of fifteen. Furthermore, a negative effect of an associated therapy (such as corticosteroid therapy) on AFP gene expression (see above) cannot be excluded.

In contrast with partial hepatectomy, acute and chronic benign liver diseases have been reported to be associated with elevated levels of serum AFP (reviewed in Taketa,1990). A correlation between the severity of the disease, as reflected by the increase in serum level of transaminase activity and the magnitude of AFP activation has been reported by some authors (Silver et al.,1974; Solinas et al.,1987), but denied by others (Czaja et al.,1987). Patients with HBsAg positive chronic liver disease display more frequent abnormalities of AFP serum concentrations than HBsAg negative patients, which has led to the suggestion that a relationship might exist between hepatitis B virus replication and AFP activation.

The significance of elevated AFP serum levels in patients with acute or chronic liver disease is unclear. It is obvious that studies based exclusively on AFP serum determinations cannot provide sufficient data to understand the mechanisms of AFP activation. The establishment of a clear correlation between the replication of hepatocytes and AFP gene activation in human liver disease would require a thorough analysis at the cellular level of the type of cells expressing AFP at the mRNA and protein levels, coupled to the study of the replicative activity of liver cells. It is interesting to note that human activated T lymphocytes have been reported to express AFP mRNA (Lafarge-Frayssinet et al.,1989). Differences in AFP serum levels between partially hepatectomized and hepatitis patients could, at least in part, be explained by the participation to increased AFP synthesis of inflammatory cells. A stimulatory effect of inflammation on AFP synthesis by hepatocytes can also be postulated.

III. AFP gene activation and hepatocyte proliferation *in vitro* :

Proliferation of isolated adult rat or human hepatocytes in primary cultures can be induced by the action of strong hepatocyte mitogens, such as epidermal growth factor (EGF), transforming growth factor α(TFG α) and hepatocyte growth factor (HGF). AFP gene activation in this *in vitro* system occurs as a very early prereplicative event, with an increase of AFP transcripts succeeding shortly to the activation of the nuclear oncogenes, c-jun, c-fos and c-myc (Tournier I. *et al.*, in press). Increased AFP secretion rate into the culture medium occurs later, during the phase of logarithmic growth, that is after the entry of hepatocytes into the S and M phase, and is maintained for some time after the decline of proliferation (Leffert et al.,1978). Thus, like during *in vivo* proliferation of hepatocytes, activation of AFP gene at the mRNA level is a very early event, largely preceeding the entry of hepatocytes into the cell cycle and AFP synthesis and secretion appears delayed in comparison with AFP mRNA activation.

IV. AFP gene activation and proliferation of transformed hepatocytes :

During chemical hepatocarcinogenesis in rats, the mechanisms of AFP gene activation appear complex. During the preneoplastic stage of azodye hepatocarcinogenesis, the main cells involved in AFP gene expression comprise 2 subsets of cells with a high proliferative activity, the oval cells and the basophilic hepatocytes (Scoazec et al.,1989) which have been shown to derive from the oval cells (Evarts et al.,1989). In these 2 cell subsets, expression of AFP mRNA is prominent, and high amount of the AFP protein are also detectable. In addition, some hepatocytes exhibit a mild increase of both nuclear and cytoplasmic mRNA, without any immunohistochemically detectable protein. This pattern of gene activation is reminiscent of the one observed in proliferating adult hepatocytes, and is presumably linked to an asynchronized proliferative response of hepatocytes consequent to toxic injury, although no direct evidence for such a relation has been provided so far. At the neoplastic stage, on the other hand, several observations suggest that expression of the AFP gene cannot be directly correlated with the proliferating activity of transformed hepatocytes : 1) expression of AFP is inconstant at the tumoral stage, and is independent of the degree of morphological differentiation ; 2) in a given tumor, there is a striking heterogeneity in the level of AFP transcripts, with a juxtaposition of positive and negative areas within the same tumor ; 3) dysregulation of AFP gene expression is also apparent in some neoplastic cells with high amount of AFP transcripts but no detectable AFP protein; 4) in some hepatoma cell lines, factors which decrease the growth rate of neoplastic cells, such as dexamethasone increase AFP synthesis (De Néchaud et al.,1976). Taken together, these data show that dysregulation of the control of cell proliferation which is a characteristic of neoplastic cells is paralleled by dysregulation of the AFP gene .

V. The oncogene connection :

AFP gene regulation appears to be linked with circumstances during which nuclear oncogenes are activated : normal liver development, liver regeneration, carcinogenesis and hepatocyte replication *in vitro*. Among nuclear proto-oncogenes, c-jun and c-fos are transcription factors which play a major role in the control of gene expression. The products of these oncogenes dimerize to form a stable transcriptional factor, AP-1, which binds with high affinity to an AP-1 binding site located on the promoter of a number of growth and developmentally regulated genes. Recently, a functional AP-1 binding site has been demonstrated on the rat AFP promoter, and AP-1 activity has been shown to positively regulate the AFP promoter *in vitro* (Zhang et al.,1991). Moreover, the AP-1 induced activation of AFP can be repressed by the glucocorticoid receptor in the presence of dexamethasone (Zhang et al.,1991). Such a mechanism of oncogene activation and glucocorticoid modulation of the AFP promoter might explain the stage specific expression of AFP. The decrease of the expression of the AFP gene after birth migh be due to the decrease of AP-1 proteins combined with a rise in corticosterone plasma levels described from the 2nd to the 3rd post-natal week in rat. C-jun and c-fos are also activated during liver regeneration, hepatocarcinogenesis and hepatocyte replication *in vitro*, paralleling the expression of AFP. Whether AP-1 activation is the main mechanism involved in AFP gene regulation *in vivo* constitutes an attractive hypothesis which remains to be demonstrated more directly.

REFERENCES

Abelev,G.I.(1971): Alpha-fetoprotein in ontogenesis and its association with malignant tumors. *Adv. Cancer Res.* 14, 295-358.

Alpert,E. & Feller, E.R.(1978): α-fetoprotein (AFP) in benign liver disease. Evidence that normal liver regeneration does not induce AFP synthesis. *Gastroenterology* 74, 856-858.

Bélanger L. et al. 1981) : Glucocorticosteroid suppression of α_1-fetoprotein synthesis in developing rat liver. Evidence for selective gene repression at the transcriptional level. *Biochemistry* 20, 6665-6672.

Bernuau D. et al. (1988) : In situ cellular analysis of α-fetoprotein gene expression in regenerating rat liver after partial hepatectomy. *Hepatology* 997-1005.

Czaja A.J. et al. (1987) : Frequency and significance of serum α-fetoprotein elevation in severe hepatitis B surface antigen-negative chronic active hepatitis. *Gastroenterology* 93, 687-692.

De Néchaud B. et al. (1976) : Effect of glucocorticoids on fetoprotein production by an established cell line from Morris hepatoma 8994. *Biochim. Biophys. Res. Commun.* 68, 8-15.

Evarts R.P. et al. (1989) : In vivo differentiation of rat liver oval cells into hepatocytes. *Cancer Res.* 49, 1541-1547.

Grisham J.W. (1962) : A morphologic study of deoxyribonucleic acid synthesis and cell proliferation in regenerating rat liver : autoradiography with thymidine-H^3. *Cancer Res.* 22, 842-849.

Lafarge-Frayssinet CH. et al. (1989) : Alpha-fetoprotein gene expression in human lymphoblastoid cells and in PHA-stimulated normal T-lymphocytes. *Biochim. Biophys. Res. Commun.* 159, 112-118.

Le Bouton A.V. (1974) : Growth mitosis and morphogenesis of the single liver acinus in neonatal rats. *Dev. Biol.* 41, 22-30.

Leffert H. *et al.* (1978) : Growth state-dependent phenotypes of adult hepatocytes in primary monolayer culture. *Proc. Natl. Acad. Sci. USA* 75, 1834-1838.

Lemire J.M.& Fausto N. (1991) : Multiple α-fetoprotein RNAs in adult rat liver: cell type-specific expression and differential regulation. *Cancer Res.* 51, 4656-4664.

Lemire J.M. *et al.* (1991) : Oval cell proliferation and the origin of small hepatocytes in liver injury induced by D-galactosamine. *Am. J. Pathol.* 139, 535-552.

Nakabayashi H. *et al.* (1989) : Transcriptional regulation of α-fetoprotein expression by dexamethasone in human hepatoma cells. *J. Biol. Chem.* 264, 266-271.

Panduro A. *et al.* (1986) : Transcriptional switch from albumin to α-fetoprotein and changes in transcription of other genes during carbon tetrachloride induced liver regeneration. *Biochemistry* 25, 1414-1420.

Petropoulos C. *et al.* (1983) : α-fetoprotein and albumin mRNA levels in liver regeneration and carcinogenesis. *J. Biol. Chem.* 258, 4901-4906.

Poliard A.M. *et al.* (1986) : Cellular analysis by in situ hybridization and immunoperoxidase of alpha-fetoprotein and albumin gene expression in rat liver during the perinatal period. *J. Cell Biol.* 103, 777-786.

Poliard A. *et al.* (1990) : Regulation of the rat α-fetoprotein gene expression in liver. Both the promoter region and an enhancer element are liver-specific and negatively modulated by dexamethasone. *J. Biol. Chem.* 265, 2137-2141.

Schmid P. & Schulz W.A. (1990) : Coexpression of the c-myc protooncogene with α-fetoprotein and albumin in fetal mouse liver. *Differentiation* 45, 96-102.

Scoazec J.Y. *et al.* (1989) : Cellular expression of α-fetoprotein gene and its relation to albumin gene expression during rat azo-dye hepatocarcinogenesis. *Cancer Res.* 49, 1790-1796.

Shiojiri N. *et al.* (1991) : Cell lineages and oval cell progenitors in rat liver development. *Cancer Res.* 51, 2611-2620.

Silver H.K.B. *et al.* (1974) : The detection of $α_1$-fetoprotein in patients with viral hepatitis. *Cancer Res.* 34, 244-247.

Solinas A. *et al.* (1987) : Alpha-fetoprotein and hepatitis B virus infection in chronic liver disease. *J. Nuclear Med & Allied Sci.* 31, 183-188.

Taketa K. (1990) : α-fetoprotein : reevaluation in hepatology. *Hepatology* 12, 1420-1432.

Tournier I. *et al.* (1988) : Cellular analysis of α-fetoprotein gene activation during carbon tetrachloride and D-galactosamine-induced acute liver injury in rats. *Lab. Invest.* 59, 657-665.

Wan Y.J.Y.& Chou J.Y. (1989) : Expression of the α-fetoprotein gene in adult rat liver. *Arch. Biochem. Biophys.* 270, 267-276.

Zhang X-K. *et al.* (1991) : Regulation of α–fetoprotein gene expression by antagonism between AP-1 and the glucocorticoid receptor at their overlapping binding site. *J. Biol. Chem.* 266, 8248-8254.

Liver Regeneration. Eds D. Bernuau, G. Feldmann. John Libbey Eurotext, Paris © 1992, pp. 123-127.

The role of growth limiting mechanisms in the regulation of liver mass and liver regeneration

Claude Nadal

CNRS – URA 1343, Institut Curie, Bâtiment 110, Centre Universitaire, 91405 Orsay, France

The existence of a growth/proliferation limiting mechanism is an old problem. Is such a mechanism partly responsible for the regulation of liver size ? It might participe in the balance of liver growth and body growth in young rats, the limitation of liver size in adult rats and the reconstitution of liver mass after partiel hepatectomy.

The problem may be approached by the search for possible inhibitory factors. The screening of various biological compounds was made by testing their activity towards hepatocyte proliferation after 2/3 hepatectomy in rat or proliferation of liver derived cell lines. Many already known biological compounds were tested. The possibility of a humoral regulation led to search for inhibitory factors in blood. The theory of chalones, a tissue or organ produces its own inhibitor, led to search for inhibitory factors in organ extracts (see review in Nadal 1979, Iype & Mcmahon 1984).

Another experimental approach would be to investigate wether there is a detectable proliferation blocking mechanism whatever the way it functions. The study of stimulations of hepatocyte proliferation which do not reduce liver mass and give unequivocal and reproducible responses make it possible to investigate what kinds of rats are responsive or not to these stimulations.

The most reliable ways to induce hepatocyte proliferation *in vivo* without reducing liver mass are stimulations of some liver metabolic activities. We will show here the results obtained with 2 of them : cytochrome P450 induction and acute inflammation.

Cytochromes P450 are a superfamily of enzymes which oxydize lipophilic compounds as a first step for their metabolism or detoxication. Substances which are substrates induce the synthesis of these enzymes. They also induce liver hypertrophy and hepatocyte proliferation. Cyproterone, an anti-androgenic steroid, is one of the most active drugs of that kind (Schulte-Herman 1974, Schulte-Herman et al. 1980).

Acute inflammation may be induced by a subcutaneous injection of irritating substance like turpentine or Freund's adjuvant. In our study we used an alkalin casein solution which is well tolerated and does not impair body growth (Nadal 1970, 1973). At least two elements of acute inflammation involve the liver : α_1 adrenergic stimulation due to stress provokes a glycogenolysis and increases cellular c-AMP, the synthesis of acute-phase proteins is induced by IL6.

We observed the effect of these stimulations in various kinds of rats. (1) Suckling rats grow rapidly, their body and liver weight double every 6 days, their relative liver weight is 3.7 %, lower than in adults, their hepatocyte proliferation is important, the labelling index (LI) is about 4 % (Nadal 1986). (2) Adult rats grow very slowly, their relative liver weight is 5 %, hepatocyte renewal and proliferation are very low and the LI is less than .1. (3) Adult rats 40 hours after 2/3 hepatectomy have already completed the first synchronized wave of proliferation and have an unsynchronized hepatocyte proliferation and a LI between 5 and 7.

MATERIALS AND METHODS

Rats were from the Wistar strain. 2/3 hepatectomy was performed according to Higgins and Anderson (1931). Cyproterone was dissolved in maize oil and given by force feeding at a dose of 100 mg.Kg^{-1}. Casein solution was : casein 3.5 g, sodium hydroxyde .3 g, H_2O 100 ml. It was injected subcutaneously at a dose of 20 ml.Kg^{-1}.

Tritiated thymidine was injected 1 hour before killing. Autoradiography was performed with histological preparations and Kodak NTB3 emulsion. Labelling index was measured by counting at least 2500 nuclei.

TABLE 1

	No treatment	Casein solution	Cyproterone
Suckling rats	3.6 ± .2	21 ± 1.4 (b)	28 ± 3 (b)
Adult rats	.08 ± .02	.6 ± .14 (a)	2.7 ± .4 (b)
Adults rats 40 hours after 2/3 hepatectomy	5 ± .7	16 ± 1.6 (b)	42 ± 3.2 (b)

Maximum LI observed after treatment of rats with either cyproterone or casein solution injection (a : $p < .01$, b : $p < .001$ versus controls).

RESULTS (Table 1)

In 10 days old suckling rats (20 g) hepatocyte proliferation was stimulated and the LI peaked 24 hours after cyproterone feeding and 20 hours after casein solution injection. It reached 5 to 7 times the normal level. So suckling rats are very sensitive to hepatocyte proliferation inducing treatments.

In two month old adult male rats (250 g) the LI rose moderately 19 hours after cyproterone feeding, approximately 10 times less than in suckling rats. After casein solution injection the LI rise was still lower.

When 2/3 hepatectomized adult rats were given cyproterone 40 hours after surgery, the LI rose to 8 times the level of hepatectomized controls 16 hours after feeding. After casein solution injection the LI rose to 3 times the control level 23 hours after injection.

DISCUSSION

These results show that some stimulations of hepatocyte metabolic activity also induce hepatocyte proliferation. Suckling rats and hepatectomized rats which have a low relative liver mass are very reactive to these stimultions, inversely adult rats are nearly unsensitive. This proliferation induced by metabolic activity could be an important way to adapt liver mass to body needs. Results obtained in adults show that a block of hepatocyte proliferation occurs when the liver reaches its adequate mass.

What is the mechanism of this block ? The stimulation of hepatocyte proliferation could need several positive factors, metabolic activity being one of them. Some of these factors could be lacking in adults and stimulations of hepatocyte metabolic activities would thus have little effect on proliferation. Conversely the block could be due to the presence of proliferation inhibitory factors. In fact, both mechanisms might coexist. Many inhibitory factors have been studied. We will summarize the characteristics of some of them which are currently under inverstigation.

βTGF has been demonstrated to have an inhibitory activity on hepatocyte proliferation in vitro (Carr et al. 1986, Strain et al. 1987). In the liver it is not produced by hepatocyte but by endothelial and Kuffer cells. After 2/3 hepatectomy its m-RNA increases and peaks 24 and 72 hours after surgery. Injection of βTGF inhibits the early proliferative response but repeated injections do not prevent liver mass reconstitution on the 5 th day after surgery (Russel et al. 1988).

Iype & McMahon (1984) and later Hugget et al. (1987), and Chapekar et al. (1989) have studied a protein extracted from the liver. Its PM is around 20-26 Kd. It inhibits the proliferation of rat liver epithelial cell lines but not the proliferation of hepatomas.

Richelt (1990) has purified a peptide from liver extracts. Its structure is Pyroglu-Asp-Ser-Gly. It decreases DNA synthesis and mitotic index in 2/3 hepatectomized mice.

A glycopeptide extracted from blood was studied by the groups of Nadal, Boffa and VanHeijenoort, Blanot, Auger. it is prepared form human α_2 macroglobuline by incubation with trypsin at the critical molecular ratio of 1/1 (Lambin et al. 1987). It is active *in vivo* and *in vitro*. *In vivo* it blocks the G.S. transition of hepatocytes in synchronized systems : the proliferation induced by acute inflammation in suckling rats, and the first wave of proliferation after 2/3 hepatectomy in adults and also in the non synchronized spontaneous proliferation of suckling rats (Nadal 1973, 1987, Nadal et al. 1981). *In vitro*, it is not active on H35 Reuber hepatoma (Fao) or Hep G_2 but is active on the WIF12-1 cell line (FAO x human fibroblast WI38 hybrid) which has a good biochemical and hepatocytic differentiation (Cassio et al. 1991). The PM is around 4000. The structure is not completely known. Its activity is destroyed by pronase, papain, and pyroglutamate aminopeptidase, not by trypsin or chyrotrypsin. It is also destroyed by association of Neuraminidase and β galactosidase (Le Rumeur et al. 1983, Auger et al. 1989). It would thus be a short peptide beginning by a pyroglutamic acid having a sugar chain necessary for activity ended by the sequence β galactosidase neuraminidase.

CONCLUSION

There is a strong experimental support for a liver growth regulation with positive and negative mechanisms. Beside growth factors, and probably in cooperation with them, stimulations of hepatocyte metabolic activities also increase proliferation and this could be an important way to adapt liver mass to body needs. When liver mass increases, a liver growth/proliferation limiting mechanism develops so that metabolic stimulations no longer result in hepatocyte proliferation.

Several inhibitory factors are presently under investigation and other will probably be found. Some of them are probably active localy, within the liver and participate in tissue and organ structure. Others might be active at the body level and participate in the regulation of liver size.

REFERENCES

Auger, G., Blanot, D., Van Heijenoort, J., Nadal, C., Gournay, M.F., Winchenne, J.J., Boffa, G.A., Lambin, P., Maes, P., and Tartar, A. (1989) : Purification and partial caracterization of a hepatocyte antiproliferative glycopeptide. *J. Cell. Biochem.* **40**, 439-451.

Braun, L., Mead, J.E., Panzica, M., Mikumo, R., Bell, G.I., and Fausto, N. (1988) : Transforming growth factor β mRNA increases during the liver regeneration: A possible paracrin mechanism of growth regulation. *Proc. Natl. Acad. Sci. USA* **85**, 1539-1543.

Carr, B.I., Hayashi, I., Branum, E.L., and Moses, H.L. (1986) : Inhibition of DNA synthesis in rat hepatocytes by platelet derived type transforming growth factor. *Cancer Res.* **46**, 2330-2334.

Cassio, D., Hamon-Benais, C., Guérin, M., and Lecoq, O. (1991) : Hybrid cell lines constitute a potential reservoir of polarized cells : isolation and study of highly differenciated hepatoma derived hybrid cells able to form functional bile canaliculi *in vitro. J. Cell. Biol.* **115**, 1397-1408

Chapekar, M.S., Hugget, A.C., and Thorgeirsson, S.S., (1989) : Growth modulatory effects of a liver-derived growth inhibitor, transforming growth factor β_1, and recombinant tumor necrosis factor α in normal and neoplastic cells. *Exp. Cell. Res.* **185**, 247-257.

Higgins, G.M., and Anderson, R.M. (1931) : Experimental pathology of the liver. 1. Restoration of the liver of the white rat following partial surgical removal. *Arch. Pathol.* **12**, 186-202.

Huggett, A.C., Krutzsch, H.C., and Thorgeirsson, S.S. (1987) : Characterization of a hepatic proliferation inhibitor (HPI) : effect of HPI on the growth of normal liver cells. Comparison with transforming growth factor β. *J. Cell. Biochem.* **35**, 305-314.

Iype, P.T., and McMahon, J.B. (1984) : Hepatic proliferation inhibitor. *Mol. Cell. Biol.* **59**, 57-80.

Lambin, P., Nadal, C., Winchenne, J.J., and Boffa, G.A. (1987) : Libération à partir de l'α_2 macroglobuline humaine d'un peptide inhibiteur de la transition G_1-S des hépatocytes *in vivo*. Rôle de la trypsine, de la thrombine et de divers agents chimiques. *C.R. Acad. Sci. Paris* **304**, 477-480.

Le Rumeur, E., Wichenne, J.J., Boffa, G.A., and Nadal, C. (1983) : Rat serum factors inhibiting the G_1-S transition in hepatocytes. II. Properties of the low molecular weight factor. *Cell Tiss. Kinet.* **16**, 333-342.

Nadal, C. (1970) : Contrôle de la multiplication et de la polyploïdie des hépatocytes du rat. Etude des perturbations de la régulation physiologique causées par l'injection de produits irritants. *Wilhelm Roux Archiv.* **166**, 136-149.

Nadal, C. (1973) : Synchronization of baby rat hepatocytes, a new test for the detection of factors controling DNA synthesis in rat hepatic cells. *Cell Tiss. Kinet.* **6**, 437-446.

Nadal, C. (1979) : Control of liver growth by growth inhibitors (Chalones). *Arch. Toxicol.*, **suppl. 2**, 131-142.

Nadal, C. (1986) : Some aspects of the regulation of hepatocyte proliferation. *Toxicologic Pathology* **14**, 349-352.

Nadal, C. (1987) : Inhibition of hepatocyte proliferation *in vivo* by a glycopeptide from rat serum. *Cell. Tiss. Kinet.* **20**, 331-341.

Nadal, C., Le Rumeur, E., and Boffa, G.A. (1981) : Rat serum factors inhibiting the G_1-S transition in hepatocytes. I. Production of a low molecular weight inhibitor by proteases or liver fractions. *Cell Tiss. Kinet.* **14**, 601-609.

Reichelt, K.L., Paulsen, J.E., and Elgjo, K. (1990) : Isolation of a growth and mitosis inhibitory peptide from mouse liver. *Virchows Archiv. B Cell Pathol.* **59**, 137-142.

Russel, W.E., Coffey, R.J., Ouelette, A.J., and Moses, H.L. (1988) : Type β transforming growth factor reversibly inhibits the early proliferative response to partial hepatectomy in rat. *Proc. Natl. Acad. Sci. USA* **85**, 5126-5130.

Schulte-Hermann, R. (1974) : Induction of liver growth by xenobiotic compounds and other stimuli. *Critical reviews in toxicology* **3**, 97-158.

Schulte-Hermann, R., Hoffman, V., Parzefall, W., Kallenbach, M., Gerhardt, A., and Schuppler, J. (1980) : Adaptive responses of rat liver to the gestagen and anti-androgen cyproterone acetate and other inducers. II. Induction of growth. *Chem. Biol. Interactions* **31**, 287-300.

Strain, A.J., Frazer, A., Hill, D.J., and Milrer, R.D.G. (1987) : Transforming growth factor β inhibits DNA synthesis in hepatocytes isolated from normal and regenerating rat liver. *Biochem. Biophys. Res. Comm.* **145**, 436-442.

Liver Regeneration. Eds D. Bernuau, G. Feldmann. John Libbey Eurotext, Paris © 1992, pp. 129-138.

Proliferative responsiveness of human hepatocytes in culture : evidence for the transitory expression of hepatotrophic factor(s) in the serum of patients with fulminant hepatitis or after partial hepatectomy

Pierre Blanc[1,4], Hervé Etienne[1], Martine Daujat[1], Isabelle Fabre[1], Jacques Domergue[2], Cécile Astre[3], Bernard Saint-Aubert[3], Henri Michel[4], Patrick Maurel[1]

[1]*INSERM U.128, CNRS, Route de Mende, BP 5051, 34033 Montpellier France.* [2]*Service de Chirurgie C, Hôpital Saint Eloi, 34059 Montpellier France.* [3]*Département de Chirurgie et Nutrition, Institut du Cancer, 34094 Montpellier France.* [4]*Service des Maladies de l'Appareil Digestif, Hôpital Saint Eloi, 34059 Montpellier, France*

SUMMARY

Human hepatocytes maintained in culture at low cell density on collagen-coated plates in a chemically and hormonally defined serum-free medium, exhibited proliferative response when stimulated with EGF (1-100 ng/mL), TGFα (1-100 ng/mL) or human serum (1-10%). The rate of DNA synthesis was increased on average 4.35 times with EGF, 5.4 times with TGFα and 6.5 times with serum from patients with fulminant hepatitis or after partial hepatectomy. In the presence of EGF, the amount of DNA and the number of cells per dish increased by 75 to 100% ($p<0.001$) and by 50% ($p<0.001$), respectively. In two patients with fulminant hepatitis, the mitotic activity of the serum was correlated with the seriousness of the hepatic failure (coma grade). In one of them, it decreased to background level after hepatic transplantation with an apparent half-life of 21 hours. The mitotic activity of the serum from hepatectomized patients reached a maximum 24 to 48 hours after surgery and returned to control level within 4 days thereafter. The magnitude of the effect was correlated with the branched amino acids to aromatic amino acids ratio, a parameter known to be related to the mass of liver resected.

INTRODUCTION

Liver regeneration is critical for the survival of patients after acute or during chronic hepatic injury (Michalopoulos, 1990; Matsumoto & Nakamura, 1991). Numerous studies have been aimed at the understanding of this phenomenon at the level of the controlling factors and their mechanism of action. Two experimental models have been used. *In vivo*, liver regeneration was induced after either partial (two third) hepatectomy or treatment of animals with hepatotoxic chemicals such as carbon tetrachloride. *In vitro*, animal hepatocytes in culture were shown to respond to mitotic agents under low cell density and special conditions of culture medium. The use of both models, either separately or in combination, allowed significant progress in the understanding of liver regeneration. Notably, several hepatotrophic factors have been identified and characterized including, epidermal growth factor (EGF) (Mc Gowan et al., 1981), transforming growth factor alpha (TGFα) (Mead & Fausto, 1989) and hepatopoietin A or hepatocyte growth factor (HPTA/HGF) (Nakamura et al., 1989; Miyazawa et al., 1989; Zarnegar & Michalopoulos, 1989). The blood level of HGF was reported to be greatly increased in patients with fulminant hepatitis and cirrhosis (Tsuboushi et al., 1989; Shimizu et al., 1991).

Recently, we developed a human hepatocyte culture system in which cell proliferation could be observed in response to EGF, TGFα, and human serum (Blanc et al., 1992). Here, we report the use of this culture system to characterize the extent and timing of the expression of hepatotrophic factor(s) in the serum of patients with fulminant hepatitis or after partial hepatectomy.

MATERIALS AND METHODS

Materials

Human recombinant EGF and TGFα were purchased from Boehringer Mannheim (Mannheim, Germany) and Sigma (Saint Louis, MO), respectively. Working solutions were directly prepared in the culture medium. Reagents for hepatocyte preparation and culture, including collagenase type IV, Ham F12, Williams E, hormones and vitamins were from Sigma. Methyl-^{3}H thymidine (specific activity 87 Ci/mmol) was from Amersham (Amersham, England).

Tissue sources and hepatocyte cultures

Lobectomy segments, from patients HTL48, FT9 and FT15, were obtained at the Centre Paul Lamarque and Saint Eloi Hospital, Montpellier and Rangueil Hospital, Toulouse, France. HTL48 was a 49y-old male with a liver metastasis from a rectum cancer (left lobe); FT9 was a 32y-old female with hepatic angioma on normal liver (right lobe); FT15 was a 31y-old female with hepatic angioma on normal liver (left lobe). Hepatocyte preparation and culture conditions were as described (Blanc et al., 1992). For the first 4H, 5% fetal calf serum was present in the culture medium (3mL per dish). The medium was then renewed and every 24H thereafter, in the absence of serum, unless otherwise indicated. The culture medium (hormonally and chemically defined, HCD) used here was that described by Isom and Georgoff (1984), except that the dexamethasone concentration was reduced to 10^{-7} M. Insulin and proline, two essential constituents for liver cell proliferation, were present at 0.6 mg/L and 32.25 mg/L, respectively.

Patients serum specimen

Serum from patients with fulminant hepatitis (FH), FH4 and FH5, was collected on admission and thereafter every day until recovery. Serum from patients who underwent partial hepatectomy (HX), HX1, HX2, HX3, HX8, HX11, HX15 and HX16 was collected before surgery (HX8, 11, 15 and 16) and thereafter every 24H for 96H. Serum was also collected from control subjects (CT), CT1-CT6 and from control/surgery patients who underwent digestive surgery without hepatectomy (CT/S), CT/S8 and CT/S9. Blood samples were collected on dry tubes and immediately centrifuged at 5000g before freezing at -80°C until use. Clinical characteristics of serum donor patients are presented in Table 1. Patient FH5 had a liver transplantation at day 0; at day -1, her coma grade was II, prothrombin level was 15% and factor V was 8%; at day 0 (day of transplantation) these parameters were respectively III, 12% and 5%; at day 4 following transplantation she was conscious, with a prothrombine at 100%.

Cell culture treatments

Treatment of cells started 12H after plating and lasted for 48 to 144H. EGF and TGFα were added to the culture medium as a 100x solution in culture medium; serum from patients was directly added to the medium at a final concentration between 1 and 10%. Culture medium and treatments were renewed every 24H.

Table 1. Clinical characteristics of serum donor patients.

Patient identification	Age	Sex	Etiology or diagnosis[a]	Treatment
HX1	77	M	MCC	left lobectomy
HX2	47	M	MBVC	left lobectomy+seg VIII
HX3	55	F	HAD	right lobectomy+seg IV
FH4	31	M	FH A	liver transplantation
FH5	21	F	FH C	liver transplantation
HX8	68	F	MCC	right lobectomy+seg IV, V
HX11	58	F	MGBC	right lobectomy+seg IV
HX15	55	F	HA	segments V and VI
HX16	68	M	HCC	segment IV
CT1	53	M	healthy subject	no
CT2	68	M	healthy subject	no
CT3	47	F	healthy subject	no
CT4	29	M	healthy subject	no
CT5	31	F	healthy subject	no
CT6	30	M	healthy subject	no
CT/S8	33	F	bowel obstruction	no hepatectomy
CT/S9	45	F	colectomy	no hepatectomy

a. MCC, metastatic colon cancer; MBVC, metastatic biliary vessel cancer; MGBC, metastatic gall bladder cancer; HAD, hepatic adenoma; FH A, fulminant hepatitis A; FH C, fulminant hepatitis C; HCC, hepatocellular carcinoma; HA, hepatic angioma.

<u>DNA synthesis</u>

Three hours before the time of assay, 12μCi of tritiated thymidine were added to the 3 mL of culture medium per dish. Cell lysate was then prepared by incubating 1.6×10^6 cells per mL of 0.5 NaOH, for 30 min. at 37°C and sonicating for 5 sec with a 100 W sonicator Sonimasse (Annemasse, France) set at 80% of maximum power. A 250μL aliquot was mixed with an equal volume of 25% trichloroacetic acid (TCA) and incubated for 10 min. at 37°C. Precipitated material was recovered by centrifugation at 10000g and washed 3 times with 10% TCA. Radiolabeled DNA was hydrolysed by incubation in 10% TCA for 30 min. at 90°C. The supernatant collected after 10000g centrifugation was mixed with 5 mL of scintillator Ready Safe Beckman (Fullerton, CA) and radioactivity was determined in a liquid scintillation counter. The rate of DNA synthesis was expressed as the radioactivity incorporated in cpm per mg of total protein.

Branched chain amino acid to aromatic amino acid ratio

Blood samples for amino acid determination in serum were collected in heparinized tubes. After protein precipitation with an equal volume of 10% (W/V) sulfosalicylic acid and centrifugation, the supernatant was stored at -80°C until analysed. Plasma free valine, leucine, isoleucine, tyrosine and phenylalanine levels were determined by reverse phase HPLC according to a method previously described (Turnell & Cooper, 1982) using a 5µm Ultrasphere ODS C18 reverse phase column (15x4.6 mm; Beckman Instruments, Palo Alto, CA) and a Varian Vista 54 chromatograph (Varian, Sunnyvale, CA).

Other assays

The nuclear labeling index was determined by autoradiography after 24 to 72H-labeling of cultures with 12µCi tritiated thymidine. Cells were counted directly within the culture dishes on previously delineated microscopic fields (4 per dish). The number of cells per field was then averaged and statistical comparison between cultures at time 0 and 72H, in absence or presence of mitotic treatment, was made according to the Student test. DNA was quantitated (in µg per dish) by fluorometry using 4',6-diamino-2-phenylindole-2-hydrochloride as the fluorochrome and calf thymus DNA as standard. Protein concentration was determined by the bicinconinic acid method of Pierce Biochemical (Rockford, ILL), bovine serum albumin being used as standard.

RESULTS

Effect of EGF, TGFα and serum from patients with hepatic failure

Human hepatocytes cultured at low density plating ($< 10^6$ cells per 60 mm dish) on collagen-coated dishes in the HCD medium were treated for 48H with 20 ng/mL EGF, 40 ng/mL TGFα, or 5% serum from patients with FH or after HX. The rate of DNA synthesis increased between 36 and 48H, reached a maximum at 48H and then returned to background level within 96H. The increase was on average 4.35 times with EGF (n=12), 5.4 with TGFα (n=6) and 6.5 with human FH or HX serum (n=9). Low level of thymidine incorporation occurred in confluent cell cultures (3.5×10^6 cell per dish). With all mitotic factors, the increase in the rate of DNA synthesis was accompanied by a corresponding increase in the mitotic index, the amount of DNA as well as of the number of cells per dish. For example, in cultures FT9 treated with 20ng/mL EGF, the mitotic index increased from 9 to 35%, the amount of DNA per dish from 5.2µg to a maximum of 8.7µg, and the number of cells by 50% after 72H. Similar results were obtained with TGFα and human serum from patients with FH or HX. In comparison, untreated cells exhibited low (if any) DNA synthesis and other mitotic responses. These results are in good agreement with previously published observations reported with animal hepatocytes (Shimizu et al., 1991; Zarnegar & Michalopoulos, 1989; Gohda et al., 1988). Our culture system offers accordingly an invaluable opportunity to investigate some aspects of human liver regeneration.

Evidence for the transitory expression of hepatotrophic factor(s) in the serum of patients with fulminant hepatitis or after partial hepatectomy

The extent of thymidine incorporation in the genomic DNA of human hepatocytes in primary cultures exposed 48 hours to 5% of serum, was used as a test to evaluate the presence and timing of expression of hepatotrophic factor(s) in the serum of patients with FH or after partial HX. For this purpose, serum from patient FH5 was collected every day from day - 1 to day + 5 (hepatic transplantation occured at day 0). Its effect on the rate of DNA synthesis was determined and compared with the effect of serum from healthy subjects of similar age. Results obtained with culture HTL48, as well as the evolution with time of the clinical and biological characteristics of patient FH5 from day - 1 to day + 5, are presented in Fig. 1. Clearly, the increase in thymidine incorporation was correlated with the seriousness of the hepatic failure: a 3.3 and 4.8-fold increase was observed with serum at day - 1 and day 0, respectively,

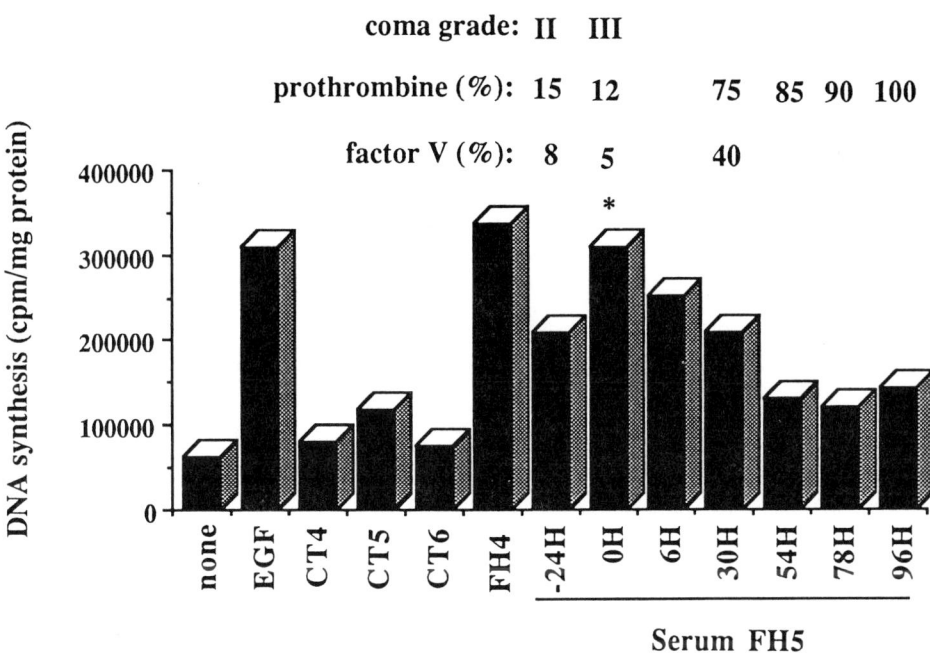

Fig. 1. **Transitory expression of hepatotrophic factor(s) in the serum of a liver transplanted patient for fulminant hepatitis.**

Hepatocytes from patient HTL48 were plated at 0.8×10^6 cells per 60mm collagen-coated dishes. The cells were then maintained 48 hours in culture in the absence or in the presence of 20ng/mL EGF or of 5% of serum from healthy subjects CT4, CT5 and CT6 or from patients FH4 (collected one day before liver transplantation) and FH5. Cells were harvested and assayed for DNA synthesis (after a 3 hour-pulse labeling with tritiated thymidine). Several samples of serum from patient FH5 were collected at: 24 hours prior to transplantation (-24H), 0 (day of transplantation), 6, 30, 54, 78 and 96 hours after transplantation. The asterisk (*) indicates the day of transplantation (0H). Clinical and biological data, concerning coma grade, prothrombin and factor V levels (in % of normal values), obtained at the times indicated are also presented.

while in the meantime, the patient passed from coma grade II to III. Notably, the stimulation of DNA synthesis returned to the background level, obtained with sera from healthy subjects, within 4 days after hepatic transplantation, in parallel with recovery of the patient. Making the hypothesis that the hepatotrophic factor(s) responsible for the stimulation of DNA synthesis was no longer produced after liver transplantation, we calculated from the semilogarithmic plot of the decay of DNA synthesis against time post-transplantation that this factor exhibited a half-life of 21 hours.

In a second series of experiments, the effect of serum collected from patients before (day - 1) and after partial hepatectomy (at day 0) from day 1 to day 4 was evaluated similarly on cultures FT9 and FT15, in comparison to those obtained with serum from patients of similar age, without hepatic pathology CT1, CT2 and CT3, or laparotomized for abdominal surgery but without hepatectomy, CT/S8 and CT/S9. The results are reported in Fig. 2. The stimulation of thymidine incorporation in response to the serum from hepatectomized patients showed a reasonable correlation with the extent of hepatectomy (Table 2): for example, right lobectomy (HX3, HX8, HX11) produced a larger effect than left lobectomy (HX1, HX2) or segmentectomy (HX15, HX16) with respect to control patients.

It has been reported that after liver resection, serum amino acids display a disturbed pattern with an increase in aromatic amino acids (AAA), Tyr, Phe and a decrease in branched chain amino acids (BCAA), Leu, Ile, Val, resulting in a decrease of the BCAA/AAA ratio correlating with the mass of resected liver (Astre et al., 1985). This ratio decreases to a minimum on the first day after hepatectomy and increases thereafter slowly, returning to its normal range within one to several months. BCAA/AAA was determined in five of the patients selected in this work, HX1, HX2, HX3, HX8, HX11. As reported in Table 2, the lower the BCAA/AAA ratio of a serum, the higher the increase in thymidine incorporation produced by this serum with respect to control. Interestingly, the serum from patients CT/S8 and CT/S9, operated for digestive pathology but without hepatectomy, did not stimulate DNA synthesis with respect to controls, before and after surgery. For hepatectomized patients, the largest stimulation of thymidine incorporation was observed at day 1 or 2 after operation (depending on the patient), the extent of stimulation decreasing thereafter with time. Finally, thymidine incorporation in response to serum at day 4 post-hepatectomy returned to the background level observed with control subjects. Thus, as observed in animals, transitory expression of a hepatotrophic factor occurs in man in response to acute hepatic failure such as fulminant hepatitis or extended hepatectomy. In the latter case, the amount of this factor seems to be related to the mass of liver resected.

DISCUSSION

Our results obtained with a human hepatocyte culture system clearly demonstrate that the expression of the hepatotrophic factor(s) in response to hepatic failure is transitory and closely related to the extent of liver damage or resection. In both patients with fulminant hepatitis, the mitotic activity of the serum was correlated with the hepatic encephalopathy (coma grade) of the patient, as observed previously by Tsuboushi et al. (1989). In hepatectomized patients, we found a rough correlation between the mass of liver resected and the mitotic activity of the serum. This correlation was examined on a more quantitative basis in five patients for whom the BCAA to AAA ratio was determined. This ratio has been shown to be correlated with the extent of hepatectomy in the rat and man (Astre et al., 1985). This is accordingly the first clear demonstration that, in man, the mitotic activity of the serum correlates with the mass of

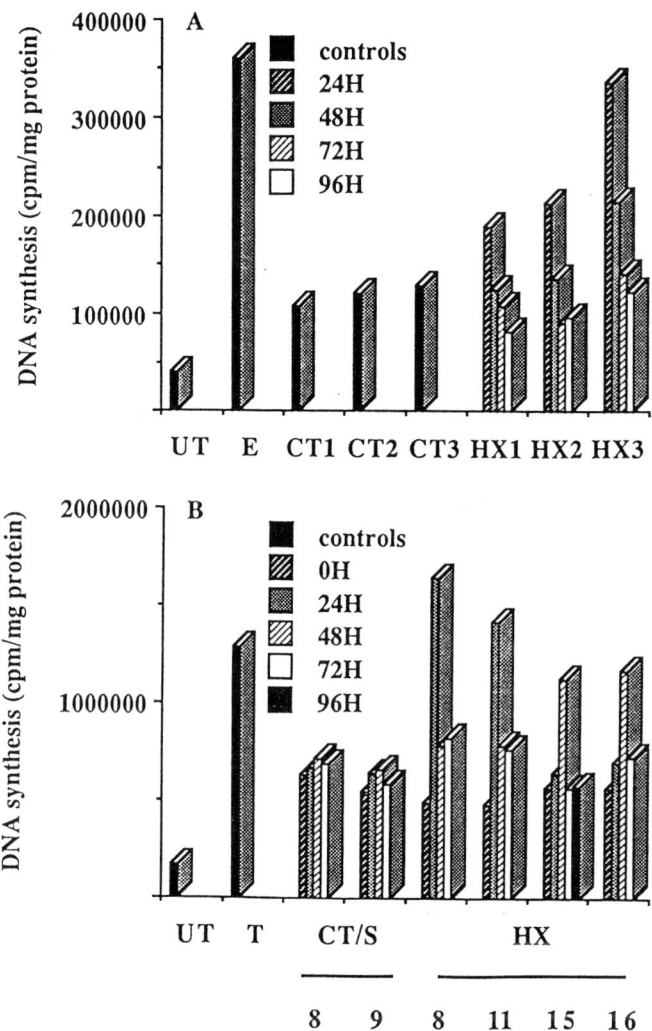

Fig. 2. Transitory expression of hepatotrophic factor(s) in the serum of patients before and after partial hepatectomy.

Hepatocytes from patients FT9 (Part A) and FT15 (Part B) were plated at 0.8×10^6 cells per 60mm collagen-coated dishes. The cells were then maintained for 48 hours in culture in the absence (UT) or in the presence of 20ng/mL EGF (E) or 40ng/mL TGFα (T) or of 5% of serum from: control patients admitted in the hospital but without hepatic pathology, CT1, CT2, and CT3; patients operated for digestive surgery but without hepatectomy, CT/S8 and CT/S9; patients subjected to partial hepatectomy, HX1, HX2, HX3, HX8, HX11, HX15 and HX16. Several samples of serum were collected from patients at time 0 (day of operation) and 24, 48, 72 and 96 hours after operation. Cells were harvested and assayed for DNA synthesis (after a 3 hour-pulse labeling with tritiated thymidine).

liver resected at hepatectomy.

In principle, analysing the mitotic activity of serum as a function of time following hepatic transplantation should provide an invaluable method of determining the half-life of the hepatotrophic factor(s). The value of 21 hours, measured with the serum of patient FH5, has to be confirmed by other methods. In hepatectomized patients, the decay in the mitogenic capacity of the serum that occurs after the maximum is close to that observed with patient FH5, the half-life here being again of the order of 24 hours. Alternatively, this decay could be interpreted as reflecting the time dependence of the release of antimitotic agents such as TGFß, which are suspected of acting in conjunction with mitotic agents to maintain the right cellular population balance (Sporn & Roberts, 1988). In fact, TGFß mRNA was shown to remain at a low level for 18-24 hours, and then to peak 72 hours after liver resection in the rat (Braun et al., 1988). In the absence of published data on the timing of expression of these various agents in man, further investigation is needed before it will be possible to understand the processes accounting for the transitory effect of serum on DNA synthesis described here.

Table 2. Mitotic activity and the BCAA/AAA ratio of serum from patients after partial hepatectomy.

Patient identification[a]	DNA synthesis[b]	BCAA/AAA ratio[c]
HX1	1.6	2.1
HX2	1.8	1.8
HX3	2.9	1.2
HX8	3.4	1.2
HX11	2.9	0.6

a. Serum samples, collected every day before and after operation for 4 days, were assayed for their capacity to increase the rate of DNA synthesis in human hepatocytes in culture (FT9, FT15) and the BCAA/AAA ratio was determined.
b. Relative increase of rate of DNA synthesis (at maximum i. e. at 24 or 48 hours) with respect to control serum (HX1, HX2, HX3) or to serum before operation (HX8, HX11).
c. BCAA/AAA ratio 24 hours after operation (normal range in healthy subjects 3.5 ± 0.5).

Several reports (Szalowski et al., 1986; Nagasue et al., 1987; Jansen et al., 1990) demonstrated using single-photon emission computed tomography that, after a 50% hepatectomy in man, the period of liver regeneration to restore 75% of the resected mass lasted between 1 and 4 months, in agreement with previous observations that the BCAA/AAA ratio returns to its normal range (3.5 ± 0.5) within one to several months (Astre et al., 1985). This appears to be rather long in comparison to the relatively short period of time during which the serum of the patient exhibits high mitotic activity (Figure 2). Two alternatives have to be considered here in discussion of this point. First, as suggested by Michalopoulos in a recent review (1990), it would appear that an extra hepatic mitotic signal is rapidly emitted, most likely HGF or HPTA. This factor was recently shown to be produced in a number of tissues including notably liver, pancreas, and Brunner's glands in the duodenum (Zarnegar et al., 1990; Tashiro et al., 1990). Its release, in response to hepatectomy, could account for the increased mitotic activity of the serum detected here 24 to 48 hours after liver resection. This factor should then stimulate the production of other mitotic agents like TGFα by the hepatocytes themselves. These agents could play their role in both autocrine and paracrine ways, so that they would not be detectable in the serum. Secondly it might be suggested that, as observed in the rat (Zajicek et al., 1989), hepatotrophic factors could be released after hepatectomy through successive mitotic waves. Interestingly, Nagasue et al. (1987) observed increased mitotic activity in the human liver, 10 and 35 days after hepatectomy. Biochemical and clinical studies aimed at a tentative clarification of this point are currently being undertaken in our laboratories.

ACKNOWLEDGMENTS

This work was supported in part by "La Caisse Nationale d'Assurance Maladie des Travailleurs Salariés".

REFERENCES

Astre, C., Saint Aubert, B., Faurous, P., Gouttebel, M.C., Collet, H., & Joyeux, H. (1985) Correlation between BCAA/AAA ratio evolution and hepatic growth after extensive liver resection in cancer patients. *Clin. Nutrition* 4, 103 (Abstract).

Blanc, P., Etienne, H., Daujat, M., Fabre, I., Zindy, F., Domergue, J., Astre, C., Saint Aubert, B., Michel, H., & Maurel, P. (1992) Mitotic responsiveness of cultured adult human hepatocytes to EGF, TGFα and human serum. *Gastroenterology.* in press.

Braun, L., Mead, J.E., Panzica, M., Mikumo, R., Bell, G.I., & Fausto N. (1988) Transforming growth factor ß mRNA increases during liver regeneration: a possible paracrine mechanism of growth regulation. *Proc. Natl. Acad. Sci. USA.* 85, 1539-1543.

Gohda, E., Tsuboushi, H., Nakayama, H., Hirono, S., Sakiyama, O., Takahashi, K., Miyazaki, H., Hashimoto, S., & Daikuhara, Y. (1988) Purification and partial characterization of hepatocyte growth factor from plasma of a patient with fulminant hepatic failure. *J. Clin. Invest.* 81, 414-419.

Isom, H.C., & Georgoff, I. (1984) Quantitative assay for albumin-producing liver cells after simian virus 40 transformation of rat hepatocytes maintained in chemically defined medium. *Proc. Natl. Acad. Sci. USA* 81, 6378-6382.

Jansen, P. L. M., Chamuleau, A.F.M., Van Leeuwen, D.J., Schipper, H.G., Busemann-Sokole, E., & Van Der Heyde, M.N. (1990) Liver regeneration and restoration of liver function after partial hepatectomy in patients with liver tumors. *Scand. J. Gastroenterol.* 25, 112-118.

Matsumoto, K., & Nakamura, T. (1991) Hepatocyte growth factor: molecular structure and implications for a central role in liver regeneration. *J. Gastroent. Hepatol.* 6, 509-519.

Mc Gowan, J.A., Strain, A.J., & Bucher, N.L.R. (1981) DNA synthesis in primary cultures of adult rat hepatocytes in a defined medium: effects of epidermal growth factor, insulin, glucagon, and cyclic AMP. *J. Cell. Physiol.* 180, 353-363.

Mead, J.E., & Fausto, N. (1989) Transforming growth factor α may be a physiological regulator of liver regeneration by means of an autocrine mechanism. *Proc. Natl. Acad. Sci. USA.* 86, 1558-1562.

Michalopoulos, G.K. (1990) Liver regeneration: molecular mechanism of growth control. *FASEB J.* 4, 176-187.

Miyazawa, K., Tsuboushi, H., Naka, D., Takahashi, K., Okigaki, M., Arakaki, N., Nakayama, H., Hirono, S., Sakiyama, O., Takahashi, K., Gohda, E., Daikuhara, Y., & Kitamura, N. (1989) Molecular cloning and sequence analysis of cDNA for human hepatocyte growth factor. *Biochem. Biophys. Res. Commun.* 163, 967-973.

Nagasue, N., Yukaya, H., Ogawa, Y., Kohno, H., & Nakamura, T. (1987) Human liver regeneration after major hepatic resection. A study of normal liver and livers with chronic hepatitis and cirrhosis. *Ann. Surg.* 206, 30-39.

Nakamura, T., Nishizawa, T., Hagiya, M., Seki, T., Shimonishi, M., Sugimura, A., Tashiro, K., & Shimizu, S. (1989) Molecular cloning and expression of human hepatocyte growth factor. *Nature* 342, 440-443.

Shimizu, I., Ichihara, A., & Nakamura, T. (1991) Hepatocyte growth factor in ascites from patients with cirrhosis. *J. Biochem.* 109, 14-18.

Sporn, M.B., & Roberts, A.B. (1988) Transforming growth factor beta: new chemical forms and new biological roles. *Biofactors* 1, 89-93.

Szawlowski, A.W., Faurous, P., Saint Aubert, B., Gouttebel, M.C., Astre, C., Collet, H., & Joyeux, H. (1986) Single photon emission computerized tomography (SPECT) for monitoring regeneration of the human liver after partial hepatectomy for secondary liver tumours. *Eur. J. Surg. Onc.* 12, 389-39.

Tashiro, K., Hagiya, M., Nishizawa, T., Seki, T., Shimonishi, M., Shimizu, S., & Nakamura, T. (1990) Deduced primary structure of rat hepatocyte growth factor and expression of the mRNA in rat tissues. *Proc. Natl. Acad. Sci. USA.* 87, 3200-3204.

Tsuboushi, H., Hirono, S., Gohda, E., Nakayama, H., Takahashi, K., Sakiyama, O., Miyazaki, H., Sugihara, J., Tomita, E., Muto, Y., Daikuhara, Y., & Hashimoto S. (1989) Clinical significance of human hepatocyte growth factor in blood from patients with fulminant hepatic failure. *Hepatology* 9, 875-881.

Turnell, D.F., & Cooper, J.D.H. (1982) Rapid assay for aminoacids in serum or urine by pre-column derivatization and reverse-phase liquid chromatography. *Clin. Chem.* 28, 527-531.

Zajicek, G., Schwartz-Arad, D., & Bartfeld, E. (1989) The streaming liver V: Time and age-dependent changes of hepatocyte DNA content, following partial hepatectomy. *Liver* 9, 164-171.

Zarnegar, R., & Michalopoulos, G. (1989) Purification and biological characterisation of human hepatopoietin A, a polypeptide growth factor for hepatocytes. *Cancer Res.* 49, 3314-3320.

Zarnegar, R., Muga, S., Rahija, R., & Michalopoulos, G. (1990) Tissue distribution of hepatopoietin-A: a heparin-binding polypeptide growth factor for hepatocytes. *Proc. Natl. Acad. Sci. USA.* 87, 1252-1256.

Liver Regeneration. Eds D. Bernuau, G. Feldmann. John Libbey Eurotext, Paris © 1992, pp. 139-145.

Liver regeneration : the surgeon's point of view

Yves Panis, Jacques Belghiti

Digestive Surgery Unit, University Paris VII, Beaujon hospital, 100 Bd Général Leclerc, 92110 Clichy, France

Several studies in man (i.e. by secondary laparotomy and repeated liver scanning) have confirmed that normal remnant liver regenerate after hepatectomy (Blumgart et al, 1971). Major liver resection in non cirrhotic patients removing 70 to 80% of the liver mass is feasible with low risk. Some authors have demonstrated that a subtotal hepatectomy as large as 90% is possible provided no underlying liver disease is present on the remnant liver (Monaco et al., 1964; Starzl et al, 1975; Baer et al., 1991).

During the last decade, progress in liver surgery has permitted to increase the resectability rate of liver tumours with low mortality and morbidity rates (Iwatsuki S. and Starzl T., 1988). Resectability rate depends in part on the skill and experience of the surgeon and some very large lesions with major vessels involvement can be resected. However, the extent of resection are not yet been clearly defined, particularly in the presence of cirrhosis.

The aim of this chapter was to deal with the recent advances in liver surgery which has permitted to improve our knowledge of liver regeneration capacity after hepatectomy and to increase resection rate, including: (a) preoperative evaluation of both tumorous and extratumorous remnant liver; (b) development of technics permitting to increase the size of the remnant liver before hepatectomy; (c) biological and morphological changes observed after hepatectomy, demonstrating the capacity of the remnant liver to regenerate; (d) analysis of carcinologic results of resection of large malignant lesion.

PREOPERATIVE EVALUATION

Imaging procedures

Resectability rate depends principally on size and location of the tumour. Progress in imaging procedures (angio CT scanner, magnetic resonnance, doppler ultrasound) has permitted to improve the definition of these parameters. Volume estimations of both tumorous and extratumorous liver can be performed by serial transverse scans of the liver at 1cm intervals (Nagasue et al., 1987). Comparison between preoperative evaluation by CT and actual measured volume of the resected specimen demonstrate a close linear relationship between the CT volumes and the actual volumes, and the average difference was within ± 3 to 5% (Heymsfield, 1979). Assesment of both normal liver and tumour volume was improved by development of three-dimensional image reconstruction system from magnetic resonnance imaging (Hashimoto, 1991) or in cirrhotic patients by a morphometrical method using a color image analyzing system (Imamura et al., 1991).

The proportion of each sector in the human liver has been estimated (± 5%) as 35% for the right posterior (segments VI and VII), 30% for the right anterior (segments V and VIII), 15% for segment IV and 20% for left lobe (segments II and III) (Stone et al., 1969). For example, 65% is allocated to right hepatectomy and 35% to left hepatectomy (Fig 1).

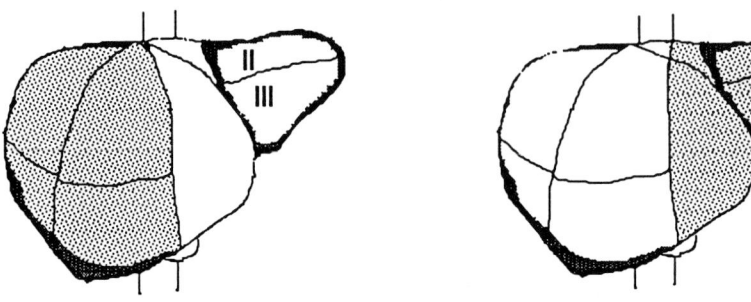

Right hepatectomy   **Left hepatectomy**

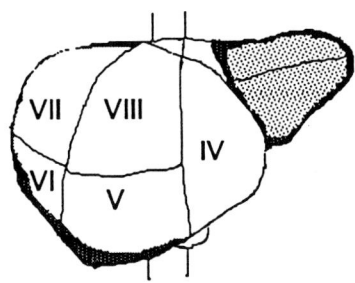

Left lobectomy

Fig. 1: The three common hepatectomies (segments according to Couinaud's classification).

Evaluation of resectability

In the absence of underlying liver disease (i.e. cirrhosis), it is estimated that extended right hepatectomy (removing segments IV to VIII) or extended left hepatectomy (segments II to V, and VIII) represents the larger resections which can be performed without risk of postoperative liver failure. After hepatectomy, the minimal remnant liver volume must range from 15 to 25% for most of the surgeons. Recently a more extensive liver resection (with respect of only dorsocranial part of segment VII and segment VI, drained by an accessory inferior hepatic vein) was reported with an uneventfull postoperative course (Baer et al., 1991).

Admitted criterias for nonresectability are thrombosis of both portal branches and discovery of a multilocular lesions involving both lobes. On the other hand, some large solitar lesions, involving inferior vena cava or main portal branch, or located into the two lobes can be resected if remnant liver is sufficient.

In case of extrahepatic biliary obstruction (i.e. Klatskin's tumor), the place of preoperative biliary drainage before resection remains still debated (Yanagisawa et al., 1988). A prospective randomized, controlled trial showed a similar postoperative complications rates between the two groups with and without drainage before surgery (Hatfield et al., 1982). However, a recent experimental study have demonstrated that cholestasis without cirrhosis altered programmed liver gene expression, inhibiting normal liver regeneration after partial hepatectomy in rats (Tracy T.F. et al., 1991). From this experimental study and from clinical reports showing a reduced mortality and morbidity rates in patients with biliary drainage (Yanagisawa et al., 1988), we advocate preoperative external biliary drainage if a major liver resection is envisaged.

Presence of associated cirrhosis

Evaluation of cirrhotic patients before hepatectomy remains difficult. Despite the use of functionnal tests as Indocyanin Green Clearance (Noguchi et al., 1990), Child's classification , if not reflecting exactly the hepatic functional reserve, is the most often used evaluation procedure. Because of the increased risk of postoperative liver failure, several authors have emphasized the risk of major liver resection in cirrhotic patients. Thus, in case of hepatocellular carcinoma complicating cirrhosis, segmentectomy or even tumorectomy were preferentially proposed (Kanematsu et al., 1984).

However we demonstrated that in low risk patients with Child A cirrhosis, more extensive resection must be proposed. Among 53 Child A cirrhotic patients operated on for hepatocellular carcinoma in our unit, a lower mortality and morbidity rate were observed after hepatectomies "réglée" than after segmentectomies (respectively 4% and 8% vs 22% and 33%). Tumorectomies were also associated with a low mortality and morbidity rates, but with a lower actuarial survival rate at 3 years than hepatectomies "réglée" (17% vs 40%).

In cirrhotic patients without preoperative liver insufficiency we found that the most important predictive factor of morbidity and mortality was a preoperative rise in aminotransferases (>100 IU/L). Morbidity and mortality rates were respectively 50% and 20% in patients with SGOT>100 IU/L and 7% and 7% in the others (Jagot et al., 1991). From this results, we conclude that preoperative evaluation of cirrhotic patients should include not only usual functionnal assessement (Child's classification) but also stigmatas of cirrhotic activities.

STIMULATION OF LIVER REGENERATION BEFORE HEPATECTOMY

Preoperative portal vein embolization

In some patients, very large resections are sometimes envisaged but finally contrindicated because of a too little remnant liver. In these cases, it was recently proposed to perform a preoperative selective embolization of the portal branch corresponding to the part of the liver that is considered for resection (Makuuchi et al., 1990). This procedure induce an hypertrophy of the non-embolized part of the liver, by stimulation of liver regeneration, and an atrophy of the embolized part. One the mechanism which could explain liver regeneration on the normal liver after controlateral portal embolization is that the same total blood flow is redistributed to a smaller mass of liver tissue, as demonstrated after major liver resections in humans, where an increase in hepatic tissue perfusion of 120% was observed (Mathie R.T., and Blumgart, 1982). However, it is now well demonstrated by experimental studies that liver regeneration after hepatectomy cannot be explain only by an increase of hepatic inflow perfusion, liver regeneration being also observed in portacavally transposed rats (Ryan et al., 1978). Theoritically, liver resection is facilitated, and the risk of postoperative liver failure diminished.

This procedure was recently reported in 54 patients with hepatocellular carcinoma complicating cirrhosis, liver metastases or cholangiocarcinoma (Makuuchi et al., 1991). Portal vein embolization was carried out via a transhepatic approach or via a transileocecal approach. The embolization materiel consisted of a mixture of gelfoam powder with urographin and gentamicin. Before portal embolization, biliary drainage was carried out in patients with cholestasis in the non-embolized part of the liver in case of extrahepatic biliary obstruction. The volume ratio between the embolized and non-embolized parts of the liver was measured by means of serial CT before surgery. Embolization was well tolerated in all patients, with mild fever in all cases and moderate rise in serum bilirubin and aminotransferases levels. Liver volumetry before surgery showed an increase in relative size of the non-embolized part of the liver of 14 % (range, 0,2-46,5%). All the patients were operated on two to three weeks after embolization and 46/54 (85%) underwent a major liver resection, with an operative mortality of 1/46 (2%). In some cases, where preoperative evaluation of liver volumes have misdiagnosed a too little remnant liver volume, or when the tumour is larger than supposed, the same result of preoeprative embolization can be obtain by a selective portal branch ligation.

POSTOPERATIVE FOLLOW-UP

Biochemical and liver function tests

Many studies have tried to evaluate the postoperative biochemical changes observed in humans after hepatectomy, but the results of these studies are difficults to analyse because of the inclusion of patients with transfusion, underlying liver disease and in some cases patients with postoperative complications. All these situations are known to modify biochemical tests after surgery (Stone and Benotti, 1989).

We explored changes in liver function tests following hepatectomy in a homogeneous group of patients without postoperative complications, and in whom no blood or plasma transfusion was given during the perioperative period (Suc et al., 1992). In this study, the postoperative changes in liver functions tests might reflect the "natural history" of hepatectomy. Our data showed: (a) a correlation between aminotransferases rise and duration of ischemia (i.e. pedicle inflow occlusion), and a fall of prothrombin time and factor V levels correlating with the weight of resected specimen; (b) a moderate g-glutamyl transpeptidase and alkaline phosphatase elevation and a rise of fibrinogen level correlating with the extent of resection at day 7; (c) changes in haemoglobin level, white cell count, platelet count, prothrombin time, factor V level and serum bilirubin level tended to return to preoperative levels by day 7; (d) for g-glutamyl transpeptidase and alkaline phosphatase, increased levels persisted for 8-12 weeks after resection.

Best indicators for liver regeneration were, firstly g-glutamyl transpeptidase and alkaline phosphatase which raised until 3 months after hepatectomy and secondly, fibrinogen level which was inversely correlated to the extent of liver resection. On the other hand, serum alphafoetoprotein is not a reliable indicator for liver regeneration after partial hepatectomy (Nagasue et al., 1987).

CT-scanning

Human liver regeneration after major hepatectomy was studied by repeated CT-scan in 17 patients (12 noncirrhotic and five cirrhotic) who underwent major liver resections (Chen et al, 1991). For non-cirrhotic liver, liver remnant volume was increased at 3 and 6 months after hepatectomy in respectively 28,4% and 48,4%; and for cirrhotic livers, in respectively 8,5% and 12,9% ($p<0,05$ vs noncirrhotic livers). Complete regeneration took about one year. Furthermore, it seemed that the greater the volume of liver resected, the greater the restoration capacity. The noncirrhotic liver that underwent right hepatectomy needed 1 year to double its postresection volume, when those which underwent only left lobectomy increased in 33% at the same date.

In patients who underwent major liver resection repeated CT scans showed: (a) a liver regeneration, correlated with the rise in alkaline phosphatase serum level; (b) a minimal liver regeneration in nonsurvivor patients who died after resection from progressive liver failure with a lower rise of alkaline phosphatase serum level; (c) a reduction of liver regeneration in patients who received chemotherapy before surgery with a lower rise in alkaline phosphatase level (Didolkar et al., 1989).

Carcinologic results

In experimental studies, after partial liver resection, the regenerating liver releases growth factors which promote hepatic mitotic activity (Naniemo et al., 1989). Theses factors have been shown to increase the growth rate of several experimental tumours after partial hepatectomy (Rozga et al., 1985). In humans, after hepatectomy for liver metastases intrahepatic recurrences occur in 30-40% of the patients and often very soon after surgery (Nordlinger et al., 1987); a higher rate of recurrence (up to 100% of the patients) is also observed for primary liver tumours complicating cirrhosis (Belghiti et al., 1991a). These recurrences, principally in case of liver metastases, could be due in part to activation by liver regeneration of cancer cells already present within the liver remnant but which remained in a dormant state until liver resection (Panis et al., 1992). Furthermore, it seemed that in patients with extensive liver resection of all but two segments of the liver as during ex-vivo liver surgery (Belghiti et al., 1991b) or less than two segments (Baer et al, 1991), intrahepatic recurrences of malignant lesions can be observed very early after surgery.

CONCLUSIONS

At present time, extensive liver resection removing up to 80% of the liver can be performed safely in specialized centers. Effective liver regeneration is observed from the remnant normal liver. The presence of cirrhosis, cholestasis, cytolysis and sequelae of chemotherapy delayed and diminish liver regeneration. New imaging procedures, including three-dimensional image reconstruction system permits careful evauation of both liver and tumorous volumes before resection. Preoperative selective portal vein embolization can be proposed before major liver resection in order to stimulate liver regeneration of the remnant liver. Best indicators for liver regeneration seems to be g-glutamyl transpeptidase, alkaline phosphatase and fibrinogen serum levels. Liver regeneration after major liver resection followed by serial CT-scan is greater in patients with normal remnant liver but is also observed in cirrhotic patients. Carcinologic results of very large liver resections remains to be evaluated, because of the possibility of tumour growth enhancement by liver regenerating process.

REFERENCES

Baer H.U., Dennison A.R., Maddern G.J., and Blumgart L.H. (1991): Subtotal hepatectomy: a new procedure based on the inferior right hepatic vein. Br. J. Surg. 78: 1221-1222.

Belghiti J., Panis Y., Farges O., et al. (1991a): Intrahepatic recurrence after resection of hepatocellular carcinoma complicating cirrhosis. Ann. Surg. 214: 114-117.

Belghiti J., Dousset B., Sauvanet A., et al. (1991b): Résultats préliminaires de l'éxérèse "ex situ" des tumeurs hépatiques: une place entre les traitements palliatifs et la transplantation. Gastroenterol. Clin. Biol. 15: 449-453.

Blumgart L.H., Leach K.G., and Karran S.J. (1971): Observations on liver regeneration after right hepatic lobectomy. Gut 12: 922-928.

Chen M.F., Hwang T.L., and Hung C.F. (1991): Human liver regeneration after major hepatectomy. A study of liver volume by computed tomography. Ann. Surg. 213: 227-229.

Didolkar M., Fitzpatrick J., Elias E., et al. (1989): risk factors before hepatectomy, hepatic function after hepatectomy and computed tomographic changes as indicators of mortality from hepatic failure. Surg. Gynecol. Obstet. 169: 17-26.

Hatfield A.R., Tobias R., Terblanche J., et al. (1982): Preoperative external biliary drainage in obstructive jaundice. Lancet ii: 896-898.

Hashimoto D., Dohi T., Tsuzuki M., et al. (1991): Development of a computer-aided surgery system: three-dimensional graphic reconstruction for treatement of liver cancer. Surgery 109: 589-596.

Heymsfield, S.B., Fulenwider T., Nordlinger B., et al. (1979): Accurate measurement of liver, kidney and spleen volume and mass by computerized axial tomography. Ann. Inter. Med. 90: 185-187.

Imamura H., Kawasaki S., Shiga J., et al. (1991): Quantitative evaluation of parenchymal liver cell volume and total hepatocyte number in cirrhotic patients. Hepatology 14: 448-453.

Iwatsuki S., and Starzl T. (1988): Personnal experience with 411 hepatic resections. Ann. - Surg. 208: 421-434.

Jagot P., Panis Y., Maignien B. and Belghiti J. (1991): Résection du carcinome hépatocellulaire sur cirrhose Pugh A: hépatectomie réglée ou simple tumorectomie. Ann. Chir. 45: 2-3 (abstract)

Kanematsu T., Takenaka K., Matsumata T., et al. (1984): Limited hepatic resection effective for selected cirrhotic patients with primary liver cancer. Ann. Surg. 199: 51-56.

Makuuchi M., Le Thai B., Takayasu T., et al. (1990): Preoperative portal embolization to increase the safety of major hepatectomy for hilar bile duct carcinoma: a preliminary report. Surgery 107: 521-527.

Makuuchi M., Kosuge T., and Lygidakis N.J. (1991): New possibilities for major liver surgery in patients with Klatskin tumors or primary hepatocellular carcinoma. An old problem revisited. Hepatogastroenterol. 38: 329-336.

Mathie R.T., and Blumgart L.H. (1982): Hepatic tissue perfusion studies during partial hepatectomy in man. Surg. Gastroenterol. 1: 297-302.

Monaco A.P., Hallgrimsson J., and McDermott W.V. (1964): Multiple adenoma (hamartoma) of the liver treated by subtotal (90%) resection: morphological and functional studies of regeneration. Ann. Surg. 159: 513-519.

Nagasue N., Yukaya H., Ogawa Y., Kohno H., and Nakamura T. (1987): Human liver regeneration after major hepatic resection. A study of normal liver and livers with chronic hepatitis and cirrhosis. Ann. Surg. 206: 30-39.

Naniemo T., Takeichi N., Hata Y., et al. (1989): Analysis of mechanism of the effect of partial hepatectomy on enhanced growth of liver cancer in rats: experimental analysis of the mechanism of recurrences after liver surgery in human liver cancers. Acta Hepatol. Jpn. 30: 889-897.

Noguchi T., Imai T., and Mizumoto R. (1990): Preoperative estimation of surgical risk of hepatectomy in cirrhotic patients. Hepatogastroenterol 37: 165-171.

Nordlinger B., Quilichini A., Parc R., et al. (1987): Hepatic resection for colorectal liver metastases: influence on survival of preoperative factors and surgery for recurrences in 80 patients. Ann. Surg. 205: 256-263.

Panis Y., Ribeiro J., Chrétien Y., and Nordlinger B. (1992): Dormant liver metastases: an experimental study. Br. J. Surg. (in press).

Rozga J., Tanaka N., Jeppson B., et al. (1985): Tumor growth in liver atrophy and growth. An experimental study in rats. Eur J. Cancer Clin. Oncol. 21: 135-140.

Ryan C.J., Guest J., Harper A.M., and Blumgart L.H. (1978): Liver blood flow measurement in the portacavally transposed rat before and after partial hepatectomy. Br. J. Exp. Pathol. 59: 111-115.

Starzl T.E., Putman C.W., Groth C.G., et al. (1975): Alopecia, ascites, and incomplete regeneration after 85 to 90 per cent liver resection. Am. J. Surg. 129: 587-590.

Stone M. and Benotti P. (1989): Liver resection: preoperative and postoperative care. Surg. Clin. North Am. 69: 383-391.

Stone H.H., Long W.D., Smith R.B., and Heynes C.D. (1969): Physiologic considerations in major hepatic resections. Am. J. Surg. 117: 78-84.

Suc B., Panis Y., Belghiti J., and Fékété F. (1992): Natural history of hepatectomy. Br. J. Surg 79: 39-42.

Tracy T.F., Bailey P.V., Goerke M.E., Sotelo-Avila C., and Weber T.R. (1991): Cholestasis without cirrhosis alters regulatory liver gene expresion and inhibits hepatic regeneration. Surgery 110: 176-183.

Yanagisawa J., Ichimiya H., Kuwano N., and Nakayama F. (1988): The role of preoperative biliary decompression in the treatment of bile duct cancer. World J. Surg. 12: 33-38.

Liver Regeneration. Eds D. Bernuau, G. Feldmann. John Libbey Eurotext, Paris © 1992, pp. 147-157.

Fulminant and subfulminant hepatitis : liver regeneration and prognosis

Jacques Bernuau

Service d'Hépatologie et INSERM U.24, Hôpital Beaujon, 100 boulevard du Général Leclerc, 92118 Clichy, France

Fulminant and subfulminant hepatitis (FSFH) is defined as acute hepatitis complicated by fulminant and subfulminant liver failure (FSFLF). From a clinical point of view, the syndrome of FSFLF is characterized by the association of jaundice, encephalopathy and marked decrease in coagulation factors activity (Bernuau & Benhamou, 1991). FSFLF most often results from widespread lesions of liver cell necrosis. The most frequent causes include acute viral hepatitis (usually due to hepatitis B virus, hepatitis D virus, hepatitis E virus and less often hepatitis A virus), drug-induced hepatitis, toxic hepatitis due to poisoning (such as acetaminophen overdose) and, rarely, auto-immune hepatitis with anti-liver and kidney microsomes antibodies (Bernuau & Benhamou, 1991). In 10 to 20% of the cases, the cause of the widespread liver cell necrosis is currently undetermined (Bernuau & Benhamou, 1991).

The overall mortality rate of patients affected by FSFH is 75% but varies from 50 to 95% according to the etiology and the patient's age (Bernuau & Benhamou, 1991). In most dying patients, a huge amount of hepatocytes is destroyed and liver atrophy may be demonstrated by X-ray computed tomography *in vivo* (Kumahara, 1989) and is a common finding at autopsy. Conversely, in most - not all - patients who survived, normal liver volume attesting full reparation of normal liver parenchyma is observed after recovery. These anatomical and histological features clearly demonstrate that liver regeneration is the cornerstone process on which critically depends the patient's outcome.

In this chapter, we will describe the various clinical and anatomical aspects of liver regeneration, as well as its serum markers and their individual prognostic value, in patients affected by FSFH. Moreover, we will present several recently reported evidence demonstrating the presence of various plasmatic factors influencing liver regeneration in patients affected by FSFH. We will then discuss the influence of some therapeutic measures on liver regeneration in these patients.

CLINICAL AND ANATOMICAL ASPECTS OF LIVER REGENERATION IN PATIENTS AFFECTED BY FSFH

In 1970, Trey and Davidson proposed to define fulminant liver failure as an acute liver disease without preexisting liver lesions and complicated by hepatic encephalopathy within 8 weeks after its clinical onset. It is now recognized that this definition encompasses rather different clinical courses which themselves depend, at least in part, on the etiology. Accordingly, in 1986, we proposed to distinguish between fulminant and subfulminant liver failure (or fulminant and subfulminant hepatitis when refering to the disease) according to the interval between the onset of jaundice and the onset of encephalopathy. Although imperfectly, these 2 profiles of the clinical course of the syndrome correlate with 2 different groups of diseases according to the etiology (Bernuau et al, 1986).

Fulminant liver failure is defined by the interval between the onset of jaundice and the onset of encephalopathy ranging between 0 and 14 days (Bernuau et al, 1986). Most frequent causes include acute viral hepatitis, acute poisoning and some cases of drug-induced hepatitis such as those due to halothane or to isoniazid. Liver cell necrosis, usually massive or submassive, is homogeneous throughout the lobule. Histological features attesting liver tissue regeneration include neocholangioles proliferation, commonly seen at the periphery of portal areas, and enlarged hepatocytes with clear cytoplasm or two-cell thick plates of hepatocytes. Death is associated with the lack of liver regeneration together with severe brain edema and acute renal failure (Bernuau & Benhamou, 1991) while survival is associated with full anatomical recovery without any sequella such as fibrosis (Karvountzis et al, 1974). These findings suggest that the patient's outcome might depend critically on which amount of liver tissue has been destroyed (Ramsoe et al, 1980; Scotto et al, 1973).

Subfulminant liver failure is defined by the interval between the onset of jaundice and the onset of encephalopathy ranging between 15 and 90 days (Bernuau et al, 1986). Most frequent causes include drug-induced hepatitis such as those due to pyrazinamide (Bernuau, personal observations), auto-immune hepatitis, the acute form of Wilson's disease and hepatitis of undetermined etiology. In few cases, the cause is acute viral hepatitis such as a recurrent bout of acute hepatitis A or acute superinfection with hepatitis D virus. Proliferation of neocholangioles is common but a noteworthy anatomical feature is the presence of regenerative, often yellowish, nodules. Because of these nodules, heterogeneous liver parenchyma suggesting liver dystrophy is a frequent finding by ultra-sound examination. Some of the nodules stick out at the liver surface. Some of them may be more than 5 cm in diameter and may be erroneously diagnosed as liver tumors. In accordance with these heterogeneous macroscopic lesions, the histological appearance of liver tissue also is heterogeneous. Massive liver cell necrosis may be seen but, most often, bridging necrosis is present (Gimson et al, 1986). Death is often precipitated by renal failure or bacterial sepsis. Survival is rare and usually associated with development of liver fibrosis or even cirrhosis. In one 35 year-old woman with subfulminant liver failure who underwent auxiliary heterotopic liver transplantation, recovery of the *native* liver was documented 6 months after transplantation (Metselaar et al, 1990).

At least theoretically, the failure of liver to regenerate in patients not surviving FSFH might be due either to the extreme reduction of the liver mass or the abnormally slowed, or even lacking, liver regeneration process, or to both. Features of liver cell proliferation as assessed by the mitotic index and the frequency of liver cells with interploid DNA values were demonstrated in liver of several patients dying from FSFH (Milandri et al, 1980). This observation suggests that, at least in some cases, the rate of liver cell destruction is a more important determinant of the patient's outcome than insufficient regeneration (Milandri et al, 1980).

SERUM ALPHAFETOPROTEIN AS A MARKER OF LIVER REGENERATION IN PATIENTS AFFECTED BY FSFH

Serum alphafetoprotein (sAFP) is a fetal serum glycoprotein the synthesis of which is repressed shortly after birth and derepressed during the course of a number of acute and chronic liver diseases (Taketa, 1990).

In patients with acute, non fulminant, viral hepatitis, sAFP usually raises during the 2nd week after the onset of symptoms. Increased values of sAFP correlate with the severity of liver cell necrosis and are more frequent in patients younger, than in those older, than 30 years (Bloomer et al, 1975). Moderate increase in sAFP level may also be observed in some cases of non viral acute hepatitis.

In patients affected by FSFH, raised sAFP levels are always associated with histological features of liver tissue regeneration (Bloomer et al, 1977; Karvountzis & Redeker, 1974) and are significantly more frequent and higher in survivors than in patients who died (Table). In one study, the difference in detectable sAFP between survivors and non survivors became significant after the 2nd day of coma (Karvountzis & Redeker, 1974). Raised sAFP levels are more frequent in HBsAg positive than in HBsAg negative patients (Karvountzis & Redeker, 1974) and in one large study correlation between sAFP levels and survival was found to be significant only in HBsAg positive patients

Table : Prevalence of raised serum alpha-fetoprotein (sAFP) in patients with fulminant or subfulminant hepatitis (FSFH)

Author (year)	Method of assay of sAFP	Patients with FSFH				HBs Ag* positive patients with FSFH	
		total number	% of those with raised sAFP all	survivors	dead	total number	% of those with raised sAFP
Opolon (1973)	immuno-precipitation	15	33	66	11	-	-
Karvountzis (1974)	counter-electrophoresis	51	56	85	38	28	67
Murray-Lyon (1976)	radio-immunoassay	64	23	48	10	8	12
Rakela (1981)	radio-immunoassay	144	-	22	-	92	33

* HBs Ag : hepatitis B surface antigen

(Rakela et al, 1981). It is also our experience that, among patients affected by FSFH, increase in sAFP is more frequent and higher in patients younger, than in those older, than 30 years and in those affected by FSFH due to acute viral hepatitis than in those with FSFH of non viral cause (Bernuau, unpublished results).

PROGNOSTIC FACTORS OF FSFH AND LIVER REGENERATION

Since liver regeneration is the cornerstone process on which critically depends the patient's outcome, it was tempting to speculate that a serum marker of liver regeneration would have a high prognostic value in patients affected by FSFH. Regarding sAFP, this hypothesis was not verified and the relationship between sAFP and the survival rate in patients with FSFH does exist, but is not infaillible (Murray-Lyon et al, 1976). In IgM anti-HBc positive patients with fulminant hepatitis B, although mean values of sAFP assayed 5 days after the onset of jaundice were 140 ng/ml and 16 ng/ml in survivors and non survivors, respectively, a multivariate analysis showed that sAFP level had only a weak *independent* prognostic value (Bernuau et al, 1986): this result indicates that sAFP level *per se* improves only slightly the prediction of the patient's outcome.

That increase in sAFP is not the most performing serum marker of successful, life-saving liver regeneration in patients with FSFH results from several reasons. First, the sensitivity of the prognostic value of raised sAFP levels is decreased by patients with FSFH who survive without increase in sAFP (Opolon et al, 1973; Karvountzis & Redeker, 1974; Murray-Lyon et al, 1976). Second, the specificity of the prognostic value of raised sAFP levels is decreased by patients who die despite raised sAFP levels. In some of these patients, extra-hepatic complications such as brain edema, bacterial or fungal sepsis, acute renal failure, severe acute pancreatitis or gastrointestinal haemorrhage are frequent findings (Bloomer et al, 1977; Murray-Lyon et al, 1976) and might have contributed to inhibit, or interrupt, the recently initiated regenerative process. In some other patients with subfulminant liver failure, ongoing liver cell necrosis persists despite raised sAFP levels and liver failure worsens while sAFP levels are declining (Bernuau, unpublished results): this observation suggests that successful, life-saving liver regeneration also requires the cessation of the destructive process of liver tissue (Gove & Hughes, 1991). Notheworthy, in patients surviving severe, non fulminant, acute hepatitis with subacute liver necrosis, sAFP reached peak levels when serum aminotransferase activity was declining (Bloomer et al, 1975).

Several studies clearly demonstrated that coagulation factors activity is the most powerful predictor of outcome in patients affected by FSFH (Bernuau et al, 1986; Harrison et al, 1990; O'Grady et al, 1989). Prothrombin time was often used (Harrison et al, 1990; O'Grady et al, 1989) but factor V - assayed on freshly sampled plasma - was shown to be the most powerful *independent* prognostic factor in fulminant hepatitisB (Bernuau et al, 1986). Recently, it was also shown to be of more accurate prognostic value than prothrombin time in patients with paracetamol induced fulminant hepatic failure (Pereira et al, 1992). Moreover, in a *prospective* study, factor V was used together with coma or severe confusion for deciding emergency liver transplantation in patients affected by fulminant viral hepatitis (Bernuau et al, 1991). Thus, since factor V is a protein manufactured *exclusively* by the liver and its raised activity in plasma is highly correlated with survival of patients affected by FSFH, one can reasonably consider this vitamin K independent coagulation factor to be an early - and currently the most powerful - serum marker of successful, life-saving liver regeneration in these patients.

EVIDENCE INDICATING THE PRESENCE OF SEVERAL CIRCULATING FACTORS INFLUENCING LIVER REGENERATION IN PATIENTS WITH FSFH

The hypothesis of the accumulation of *toxic inhibitors* of liver regeneration in plasma of patients affected by FSFH roughly paralleled the assumption that the accumulation of various substances might be toxic for the brain and responsible, at least in part, of hepatic encephalopathy. Plasma from patients with FSFH was shown to be toxic for rabbit hepatocytes (Hughes et al, 1976) and various compounds that accumulate in plasma in patients with encephalopathy due to FSFH - such as ammonia, octanoate and mercaptans - induced depression of liver thymidine kinase activity and of the incorporation of 3H-thymidine into liver DNA after they were injected into rats recently submitted to partial hepatectomy (Zieve et al, 1985). Serum from patients with FSFH was found to inhibit DNA synthesis in hepatocytes of regenerating rat livers 24 hours after partial hepatectomy (Gove et al, 1982). Similar liver DNA inhibition was found again when whole rats were injected with serum from patients with FSFH at least 20 hours, but not earlier, after partial hepatectomy indicating that the injected serum did not inhibit the initiation of liver regeneration (Yamada et al, 1990).

Other experiments demonstrate the presence of circulating stimulating factors of liver regeneration in patients affected by FSFH. Serum and plasma sampled in such comatose patients stimulate DNA synthesis in adult rat hepatocytes in primary culture (Gohda et al, 1986; Nakayama et al, 1985). More recently, human hepatocyte growth factor (hHGF) was purified and partially characterized from plasma of a patient with FSFH (Gohda et al, 1988). The growth-promoting activity of serum or plasma of Japanese patients with FSFH was 16 times higher than that of a normal serum, was *not* related to the patient's outcome but was closely related to the clinical severity of hepatic coma: the activity increased while the coma developed and decreased when the coma improved in survivors (Tsubouchi et al, 1989). Recently, sera from 2 French patients with fulminant hepatitis were shown to increase 4-6 times the rate of DNA synthesis of cultured *human* hepatocytes (Blanc et al, 1992). The precise role of hHGF and other substances stimulating liver regeneration in patients with FSFH is still unclear, but could be mainly to amplify liver regeneration shortly after its initiation (Gove & Hughes, 1991).

THERAPEUTIC MEASURES AND LIVER REGENERATION IN PATIENTS WITH FSFH

No medical treatment is known to induce or to stimulate liver regeneration in man. Since none of the numerous treatments proposed before the era of emergency liver transplantation improve the survival rate of patients affected by FSFH (Bernuau & Benhamou, 1991), it can be assumed that none of them influence favourably liver regeneration. Although infusion of insulin and glucagon was reported to be beneficial on fulminant murine hepatitis (Farivar et al, 1976), it failed both to stimulate liver regeneration and to improve survival in patients with FSFH (Harrison et al, 1990).

Restricted use of drugs is especially recommended in patients affected by FSFH because of the risks of their excessive effects due to the failure of the liver to metabolize them adequately (Bernuau & Benhamou, 1991). Another risk which is often neglected is that of drug-induced impairment of liver regeneration. Corticosteroids (EASL Trial Committee, 1979) and interferon (Sanchez-Tapias et al, 1987) which were shown not to improve, and even worsen (EASL Trial Committee, 1979), the survival rate of patients with FSFH, were also shown to be deleterious for liver regeneration in rat (Tsukamoto & Kojo, 1989) and in mice (Frayssinet et al, 1973), respectively. Any substance which alters, or interfers with, DNA synthesis must be avoided in patients affected by FSFH.

REFERENCES

Bernuau, J., Rueff, B., and Benhamou, J.P. (1986): Fulminant and subfulminant liver failure: definitions and causes. *Semin. Liver Dis.* 6, 97-106.

Bernuau, J., Goudeau, A., Poynard, T., Dubois, F., Lesage, G., Yvonnet, B., Degott, C., Bezeaud, A., Rueff, B., and Benhamou, J.P. (1986): Multivariate analysis of prognostic factors in fulminant hepatitis B. *Hepatology* 6, 648-651.

Bernuau, J., and Benhamou, J.P. (1991): Fulminant and subfulminant liver failure. In *Oxford Textbook of Clinical Hepatology*, eds. N. McIntyre, J.P. Benhamou, J. Bircher, M. Rizzetto and J. Rodés, pp. 921-942. Oxford: Oxford University Press.

Bernuau, J., Samuel, D., Durand, F., Saliba, F., Bourlière, M., Adam, R., Gugenheim, J., Castaing, D., Bismuth, H., Rueff, B., Erlinger, S., and Benhamou, J.P. (1991): Criteria for emergency liver transplantation in patients with acute viral hepatitis and factor V (FV) below 50% of normal: a prospective study. *Hepatology* 14, 49A (abstract 6).

Blanc, P., Etienne, H., Daujat, M., Fabre, I., Zindy, F., Domergue, J., Astre, C., Saint Aubert, B., Michel, H., and Maurel, P. (1992): Mitotic responsiveness of cultured adult human hepatocytes to epidermal growth factor, transforming growth factor α, and human serum. *Gastroenterology* 102, 1340-1350.

Bloomer, J.R., Waldmann, T.A., McIntire, K.R. and Klatskin, G. (1975): Relationship of serum alphafetoprotein to the severity and duration of illness in patients with viral hepatitis. *Gastroenterology* 68, 342-350.

Bloomer, J.R., Waldmann, T.A., McIntire, K.R. and Klatskin, G. (1977): Serum alphafetoprotein in patients with massive hepatic necrosis. *Gastroenterology* 72, 479-482.

Eleftheriou, N., Heathcote, J., Thomas, H.C., and Sherlock, S. (1977): Serum alphafetoprotein levels in patients with acute and chronic liver disease. Relation to hepatocellular regeneration and development of primary liver cell carcinoma. *J. clin. Path.* 30, 704-708.

EASL Trial Committee (N. Tygstrup & E. Juhl) (1979): Randomised trial of steroid therapy in acute liver failure. *Gut* 20, 620-623.

Farivar, M., Wands, J.R., Isselbacher, K.J., and Bucher, N.L.R. (1976): Effect of insulin and glucagon on fulminant murine hepatitis. *N. Engl. J. Med.* 295, 1517-1519.

Frayssinet, C., Gresser, I., Tovey, M., Lindahl, P. (1973): Inhibitory effect of potent interferon preparations on the regeneration of mouse liver after partial hepatectomy. *Nature* 245, 146-147.

Gimson, A.E.S., O'Grady, J., Ede, R.J., Portmann, B., and Williams, R. (1986): Late onset hepatic failure: clinical, serological and histological features. *Hepatology* 6, 288-294.

Gohda, E., Tsubouchi, H., Nakayama, H., Hirono, S., Takahashi, K., Koura, M., Hashimoto, S., and Daikuhara, Y. (1986): Human hepatocyte growth factor in plasma from patients with fulminant hepatic failure. *Exp. Cell Res.* 166, 139-150.

Gohda, E., Tsubouchi, H., Nakayama, H., Hirono, S., Sakiyama, O., Takahashi, K., Miyazaki, H., Hashimoto, S., and Daikuhara, Y. (1988): Purification and partial characterization of hepatocyte growth factor from plasma of a patient with fulminant hepatic failure. *J. Clin. Invest.* 81, 414-419.

Gove, C.D., Hughes, R.D., and Williams, R. (1982): Rapid inhibition of DNA synthesis in hepatocytes from regenerating livers by serum from patients with fulminant hepatic failure. *Br. J. Exp. Pathol.* 63, 547-553.

Gove, C.D., Hughes, R.D. (1991): Liver regeneration in relationship to acute liver failure. *Gut* Supplement S92-S96.

Harrison, P.M., Hughes, R.D., Forbes, A., Portmann, B., Alexander, G.J.M., and Williams, R. (1990): Failure of insulin and glucagon infusion to stimulate liver regeneration in fulminant hepatic failure. *J. Hepatol..* 10, 332-336.

Harrison, P.M., O'Grady, J.G., Keays, R.T., Alexander, G.J.M., and Williams, R. (1990): Serial prothrombin time as prognostic indicator in paracetamol induced fulminant hepatic failure. *Br. Med. J.* 301, 964-966.

Hughes, R.D., Cochrane, M.G., Thompson, A.D., Murray-Lyon, I.M., and Williams, R. (1976): The cytotoxicity of plasma from patients with acute hepatic failure to isolated rabbit hepatocytes. *Br. J. Exp. Pathol.* 57, 348-353.

Karvountzis, G.G., Redeker, A.G.(1974): Relation of alphafetoprotein in acute hepatitis to severity and prognosis. *Ann. Intern. Med.* 80, 156-160.

Karvountzis, G.G., Redeker, A.G., and Peters, R.L. (1974): Long term follow-up studies of patients surviving fulminant viral hepatitis. *Gastroenterology* 67, 870-877.

Kumahara, T., Muto, Y., Moriwaki, H., Yoshida, T., and Tomita, E. (1989): Determination of the integrated CT number of the whole liver in patients with severe hepatitis: as an indicator of the functional reserve of the liver. *Gastroenterol Jpn* 24, 290-297.

Metselaar, H.J., Hesselink, E.J., De Rave, S., Ten Kate, F.J.W., Lameris, J.S., Groenland, T.H.N., Reuvers, C.B., Weimar, W., Terpstra, O.T., Schalm, S.W. (1990): Recovery of failing liver after auxiliary heterotopic transplantation. *Lancet* 335, 1156-1157 (letter).

Milandri, M., Gaub, J., Ranek, L.(1980): Evidence for liver cell proliferation during fatal acute liver failure. *Gut* 21, 423-427.

Murray-Lyon, I.M., Orr, A.H., Gazzard, B., Kohn, J. and Williams, R. (1976): Prognostic value of serum alphafetoprotein in fulminant hepatic failure including patients treated by charcoal haemoperfusion. *Gut* 17, 576-580.

Nakayama, H., Tsubouchi, H., Gohda, E., Koura, M., Nagahama, H., Yoshida, Y., Daikuhara, Y. , and Hashimoto, S., (1985): Stimulation of DNA synthesis in adult rat hepatocytes in primary culture by sera from patients with fulminant hepatic failure. *Biomed. Res.* 6, 231-237.

O'Grady, J.G., Alexander, G.J.M., Hayllar, K.M., and Williams, R. (1989): Early indicators of prognosis in fulminant hepatic failure. *Gastroenterology* 97, 439-445.

Opolon, P., Hirsch-Marie, H., Gateau, Ph., Caroli, J. (1973): Apparition d'alpha-I-fœtoprotéine circulante au cours de l'atrophie aiguë du foie. Résultats préliminaires. *Ann. Méd. interne* 124, 883-888.

Pereira, L.M.M.B., Langley, P.G., Hayllar, K.M., Tredger, J.M., and Williams, R. (1992): Coagulation factor V and VIII/V ratio as predictors of outcome in paracetamol induced fulminant hepatic failure: relation to other prognostic indicators. *Gut* 33, 98-102.

Rakela, J., Alpert, E., Mosley, J.W. and Acute Hepatic Failure Study Group (1981): Serum alphafetoprotein in relation to prognosis in acute hepatic failure. *Hepatology* 1, 539 (abstract 49B).

Ramsoe, K., Andreasen, P.B., and Ranek, L. (1980): Functioning liver mass in uncomplicated and fulminant acute hepatitis. *Scand. J. Gastroenterol.*, 15, 65-72.

Sanchez-Tapias, J.Ma., Mas, A., Costa, J., Bruguera, M., Mayor, A., Ballesta, A.M., Compernolle, C., and Rodés, J. (1987): Recombinant alpha 2c-interferon therapy in fulminant hepatitis. *J. Hepatol.* 5, 205-210.

Scotto, J., Opolon, P., Eteve, J., Vergoz, D., Thomas, M., and Caroli, J. (1973): Liver biopsy and prognosis in acute liver failure. *Gut* 14, 927-933.

Taketa,.K. (1990): Alphafetoprotein: reevaluation in hepatology. *Hepatology* 12, 1420-1432.

Tsubouchi, H., Hirono, S., Gohda, E., Nakayama, H., Takahashi, K., Sakiyama, O., Miyazaki, H., Sugihara, J., Tomita, E., Muto, Y., Daikuhara, Y. and Hashimoto, S. (1989): Clinical significance of human hepatocyte growth factor in blood from patients with fulminant hepatic failure. *Hepatology* 9, 875-881.

Tsukamoto, I., and Kojo, S. (1989): Effect of glucocorticoid on liver regeneration after partial hepatectomy in the rat. *Gut* 30, 387-390.

Yamada, H., Gove, C.D., Hughes, R.D., and Williams, R. (1990): Effects of fulminant hepatic failure serum on hepatic DNA synthesis in normal;and partially hepactectomized rats. *Eur. J. Gastroenterol. Hepatol.* 2, 483-488.

Zieve, L., Shekelton, M., Lytfogt, C., and Draves, K. (1985): Ammonia, octanoate and a mercaptan depress regeneration of normal rat liver after partial hepatectomy. *Hepatology* 5, 28-31.

Author index

Appasamy R., 85
Astre C., 129

Balabaud C., 29
Belghiti J., 139
Bernard P., 29
Bernuau D., 117
Bernuau J., 147
Bioulac-Sage P., 29
Blanc P., 129
Bréchot C., 49, 103

Cariani E., 103
Carles J., 29
Charlotte F., 39
Chenivesse X., 49

Daujat M., 129
Domergue J., 129
Dubuisson L., 29

Etienne H., 129

Fabre I., 129
Fausto N., 1, 77
Feldmann G., 7, 117

Glaise D., 61
Guguen-Guillouzo C., 61

Henglein B., 49

Lamas E., 49, 103
Lasserre C., 103
Le Bail B., 29
Lefebvre P., 29
Loyer P., 61

Maurel P., 129
Meijer L., 61
Michalopoulos G.K., 85
Michel H., 129

Nadal C., 123

Panis Y., 139

Rosenbaum J., 39

Saint Aubert B., 129
Scoazec J.Y., 17, 117
Sobczak J., 71

Tournier I., 117

Wang J., 49

Zarnegar R., 85
Zindy F., 49, 103

Key word index

acute inflammation, 4, 72, 119, 123-125
albumin, 22, 108
alcoholic liver disease, 9, 11, 40, 41
alpha-fetoprotein, 22, 23, 81, 111, 112, 113, **117-122**, 142, 149
aminoacids, 2, 134
apoptosis, 1, 22

benign liver tumor, 30, 35, 80, 105, 108
bile duct cells, 20-23
bromodeoxyuridine, **9-11**, 40, 44, 55

c-fos, 21, 63, 66, 67, **71-76**, 121
c-jun, 63, 66, 67, **71-76**, 121
c-myc, 21, 50, 63, 66, 67, **71-76**, 81, 82, 93
c-ras, 21, 67, **71-76**, 93
cell cycle, 2, 5, 7,12, 49, 52, 62, 66, 93
cirrhosis, 9, 11, 12, 36, 39, 40, 50, 92, 105, 108, 112, 130, 141-143, 149-153
cyclins (and cyclin associated proteins), **49-59**, 62, 65, 66

DNA polymerase α, 11, 12
DNA synthesis, 2, 4, 89, 44, 52, 62, 63, 72, **78-80**, 88, 90, 91, 118, 119, 131, 132, 152, 153

endothelial cell, 29, 34, 36, 42, 86, 110, 125
epidermal growth factor, 4, 35, 52, 62, 77-79, 120, 129, 132
epidermal growth factor receptor, 79-82
extracellular matrix, 5, 31, 33, 35, 41, 42

fetal liver, 4, 78, 103, 106, 108, 112, 117, 118
fulminant hepatitis, 12, 36, 93, 130, 132-134, **147-157**

H3 histone mRNA, 12
hepatic lobule, 8, 23, 39, 40, 80, 106, 117, 118, 148
hepatitis B virus, 49, 50, 110, 111, 119, 147, 149, 151, 152
hepatocarcinogenesis, 22, 50, 81, 120
hepatocarcinoma, 11, 12, 35, 49, 50-52, 80, 81, 105, 106, 108, 109, 111-113, 141-143
hepatocyte culture, 8, 10, 52, 54, 63, 67, 78, 81, 88, 110, 120, 130

hepatocyte growth factor, 4, 30, 31, 35, 44, 62, **84-101**, 120, 130, 137, 152

inhibitory factors, 4, 5, **123-127**, 152
insulin-like growth factor I, 41
insulin-like growth factor II, 81, **103-113**

Ki 67 nuclear antigen, 12
Kupffer cell, 29, 32, 36, 41, 86, 110, 125

liver development, 4, 78, 103, 108, 112, 117, 118
liver regeneration (models), 2, 30, 32, 33, 39, 40, 49, 90, 118, 119
liver stem cells, **19-23**
liver transplantation, 1, 149, 152

mitosis, 7, 40, 62-65

norepinephrine, 90, 91

oval cells, 21-23, 119, 120

p-53, 21, 67, **71-76**
partial hepatectomy, 1, 4, 10, 29-34, 44, 49, 52, 62, 65, 71-73, 78, 79, 89, 90, 118, 123, 124, 131, 134-137, 139, 143, 152

perisinusoidal cell (Ito cell), 10, 29, 36, **39-48**, 86, 110
platelet derived growth factor, 40-42, 62
proliferating cell nuclear antigen, 12

retinoblastoma gene, 5, 72

stem cells, **17-19**

transforming growth factors, 4, 5, 30, 31, 35, 40, 41, 44, 62, **77-84**, 91, 120, 125, 129, 132
transgenic mice, 80, 81, 113
tritiated thymidine, 8, 21, 39, 40, 52, 63-65, 80, 119, 124, 132, 134, 152

LOUIS-JEAN
avenue d'Embrun, 05003 GAP cedex
Tél. : 92.53.17.00
Dépot légal : 495 — Juillet 1992
Imprimé en France